THE
Red Yeast Rice
CHOLESTEROL
SOLUTION

THE
Red Yeast Rice
CHOLESTEROL
SOLUTION

❖

Maureen Keane

BESTSELLING AUTHOR OF
Juicing for Life AND
What to Eat if You Have Cancer

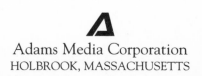

Adams Media Corporation
HOLBROOK, MASSACHUSETTS

Published by
Adams Media Corporation
260 Center Street, Holbrook, MA 02343

ISBN: 1-58062-248-8

Printed in Canada.

J I H G F E D C B A

Library of Congress Cataloging-in-Publication Data
available from the publisher.

This publication is designed to provide accurate and authoritative information
with regard to the subject matter covered. It is sold with the understanding
that the publisher is not engaged in rendering professional medical advice. If
assistance is required, the services of a competent professional person should
be sought.

*This book is available at quantity discounts for bulk purchases.
For information, call 1-800-872-5627.*

Visit our home page at http://www.adamsmedia.com

Contents

Acknowledgements

I would like to thank all those who graciously shared their information on red yeast rice with me, including: Pharmanex, Robin Gray—Dr. Chang's executive assistant, and Richard Zhang of Rich Nature Labs. I would also like to thank those who took the time to talk with me: Dr. Joseph Chang, Ph.D., the vice president of clinical affairs at Pharmanex, Inc., Dr. James Eitner of Maricopa County Public Health, and Angela Howard and Brian Hughes of Pharm N Seas.

Thanks to Sydney Harriet—my agent—for his help and to Paula Lee at Adams Media for allowing me to bring my idea to print.

I would like to thank my husband who suffered silently as his wife wrote a book leaving him to entertain fourteen out-of-town relatives. Finally, I would like to thank all my house guests who put up with an absent host.

Introduction

As a nutritionist I know how frustrating it can be to counsel people with high cholesterol. Some respond readily to a low-fat diet. For others, diet and exercise are just not enough. No matter what they do or how hard they try, their cholesterol levels refuse to budge. Until now, all nutritionists such as myself could do was offer supplements such as garlic pills, fish oil, and fiber supplements. Finally, we now have an effective and safe treatment.

Notice I say treatment—not cure. Yes, red yeast rice is safe. Yes, red yeast rice is effective. But it is not a cure or a magic pill or potion. It is simply an effective natural treatment with an impressive amount of science behind it. In order for this supplement to work it must be accompanied by a Step I diet. You simply cannot keep shoveling in saturated fat and expect your heart to stay healthy. No amount of red yeast rice can make up for a poor diet and lack of exercise. So this book is not just about red yeast rice, it is also about food and diet.

HOW TO USE THIS BOOK

In Chapters 1 though 5 you will find facts about red yeast rice, atherosclerosis, plaque, and cholesterol. These chapters explain what cholesterol is and what all those letters and numbers on your cholesterol test mean, how red yeast rice works, and the research that proves it does work, as well as other supplements you can try along with your diet. In the middle chapters you will find the red yeast rice diet and instructions on how to take the supplement. If you cannot find red yeast rice in your local health food store, turn to the back of the book for mail order sources.

The last few chapters will help you to personalize the red yeast rice diet to fit your needs. Here you will find instructions on how to evaluate your diet, blood pressure, and weight, understand your cholesterol test results, and assess your cardiovascular risk factors. Chapter 9 will help you to tweak your diet if you have special needs.

I first read about red yeast rice when I came across Dr Heber's UCLA study while browsing through the *Journal of Clinical Research*. I was very impressed with the research that had been done on this supplement. The excitement turned to frustration when I discovered that most of the allopathic and naturopathic physicians I knew had never heard of it. Even at my alma mater—Bastyr University—queries about red yeast rice drew only blank stares. The problem is that red yeast rice is so new most physicians aren't even aware it exists. Do your doctor a favor and bring a copy of this book on your next visit so he can read Chapter 5.

If you have a red yeast rice success story that you would like to share, please send it to me care of my publisher. If you have found a good red yeast rice supplement that is not on my list, let me know that and I will add it to future editions of this book.

1

The History
of Red Yeast Rice

The idea that food is linked to good health is not a new concept. It has been known since ancient times that foods can have medicinal effects. This is the basis of the traditional Chinese saying that food and medicine are from the same source. Hippocrates also championed this philosophy in 400 B.C. when he said, "Let food be your medicine and medicine be your food." For a while we forgot how important our food supply was to our health as we concentrated on the wonders of modern drugs and surgery. But drugs and other medical wonders will only do so much, and we have found that many of today's modern illnesses respond miraculously to the simple therapy of wholesome food. So as the twenty-first century begins we find that we have come full circle, as modern scientists and physicians rediscover and embrace Hippocrates's ancient philosophy. If you read the papers or watch TV, you can't help but be aware of all the new findings about the health-giving properties of whole foods. Hardly a week passes without word of some new discovery.

Garlic is such an example; it is practically a medicine chest in a bulb. Who would think that such a common seasoning could function as an antibiotic, blood thinner, cancer preventative, and immune enhancer? Some foods, such as ginger, have been tested against drugs and found to be as good or better. For example, ginger root powder was shown to be as good as or better than Dramamine, an over-the-counter drug for preventing motion sickness. In some instances soy isoflavones have been found to be an acceptable replacement for hormone replacement therapy in postmenopausal women.

WHOLE FOODS

We are going to use the term "whole foods" quite a bit in this book, so let's take a few minutes to discuss exactly what it means. Whole foods are foods that are whole. That is, no one part has been removed from the food and it has been only minimally processed and is in much the same form as nature made it. A good example of a whole food is whole grains. The wheat berry in its whole state contains: a layer of bran—an insoluble fiber coating that has many health benefits including the regulation of digestion; the germ—which contains the oils, the majority of the grain's vitamin, mineral, and phytonutrient content; and the core—which contains the carbohydrate, protein, and soluble fiber. When wheat is refined, both the germ and the bran are removed. The result is white flour, which is then enriched—some of the vitamins are added back. The result however is a far cry from the whole food.

Whole foods are vastly superior in both taste and nutrition. Your heart needs all of a food—all of its nutrients, vitamins, and fiber. A whole foods diet is one that avoids refined foods such as white flour and bread, white rice, white sugar—you get the idea. Think brown instead—brown bread, brown flour, and brown rice.

A whole food diet also avoids overly processed foods. These are the packaged, precooked, prepared, preserved, ready-to-eat type foods. They are often full of artificial flavorings and colors, preservatives, and salt and are overly cooked so that fragile vitamins are lost and overly refined so that phytonutrients and fiber are lost. Just look at the ingredient label to see how many chemicals have been added.

What makes whole foods so good for you? In the recent past it was believed that food provided only the proteins, carbohydrates, fats, vitamins, and minerals necessary for energy production and the growth and maintenance of tissue. Only health "nuts" considered food to be anything more. Today we know better. Food is more than just a tasty receptacle for vitamins and minerals. It contain numerous substances that bring additional and sometimes unexpected health benefits.

Some foods with little traditional nutrient value (no protein and few vitamins and minerals) can have a substantial effect on health. Look at the apple. It contains sugar, few vitamins, and little minerals, but when big apple eaters were compared with those who ate few or no apples it was found that the apple eaters had less upper respiratory infections and in general less tension and sickness. If these active agents in apples are not vitamins or minerals, what are they?

PHYTONUTRIENTS

In the case of apples, one active agent is thought to be the polyphenols. When you put polyphenols from foods in a test tube with viruses, the viruses are killed. Another agent is glutathione, a powerful antioxidant compound. Polyphenols and glutathione are only a few of the hundreds of health-promoting food components found in plants called phytonutrients or plant nutrients (phyto means plant). You will see the prefix "phyto" later in the book when we talk about phytosterols (plant sterols) and phytoestrogens (plant estrogens).

Since a plant cannot simply pull up its roots and walk or run away from an animal, it has to have some method of communicating or protecting itself. It does this through the use of chemicals. Chemicals with odors entice animals to eat the seed-bearing parts of plants such as fruit. The animals then aid in the spreading and fertilizing of the new plants. Color pigments attract insects that aid in pollination. Other chemicals impart a bitter or otherwise unpalatable taste that protects the plant from being eaten. Some plants can even secrete phytohormones that may act as a kind of birth control to prevent herds from over grazing and destroying whole fields. However, when humans eat these compounds not only do they make the food item attractive and palatable, they also make it healthier. These compounds actually prevent many diseases and can aid in the treatment of some.

Fruits and vegetables get their bright colors from pigments. Pigments often have value beyond that of imparting hue. The orange carotenes found in carrots and cantaloupe, the yellow flavonoids found in lemons and oranges, and the red anthocyanins found in cherries and cranberries all act as antioxidants and in that role aid in the prevention and treatment of cancer and heart disease. *Monascus purpureus*—a red yeast—produces several red pigments that are related to its cholesterol-lowering abilities. Odiferous chemicals, such as the sulfur compounds found in garlic, onions, and leeks, have antibacterial, antiplatelet, and lipid-lowering effects. Phytonutrients are also not limited to plants. They are also produced by microbes such as bacteria, mold, and yeast. For example, all three produce HMG-CoA reductase inhibitors— substances that prevent the enzyme HMG-CoA reductase from making cholesterol.

FUNCTIONAL FOODS

In 1989, the phrase *designer foods* was coined to describe foods that contained biologically active chemicals that reduced cancer risk. A few years later the term *nutraceuticals* was used to describe foods that provided medical or health benefits, in other words, foods that contained health-giving phytonutrients. Most recently, the Institute of Medicine of the U.S. National Academy of Sciences defined *functional* foods as those that "encompass potentially healthful products" including "any modified food or food ingredient that may provide a health benefit beyond the traditional nutrients it contains."

Functional foods are one of the fastest growing segments of the food industry. The current U.S. market for functional foods has been calculated to be between 7.5 billion to 9 billion with the potential markets estimated to be 250 billion dollars. Functional foods that are suspected of effecting cholesterol levels include herbs such as hawthorn (*Crataegus oxyacantha*), seeds such as psyllium, and grains such as amaranth. Red yeast rice is but one of an estimated 3,000 varieties of functional food products on the market in China.

TRADITIONAL CHINESE MEDICINE

In traditional Chinese medicine (TCM), functional foods or health foods are foods that maintain and improve health status, prevent disease, and help in treating disease and facilitating rehabilitation. In a recent paper entitled "Eastern Perspective on Functional Foods," Dr. Weng, from the College of Traditional Chinese Medicine in Beijing said this:

> In TCM food and medicine are of equal importance
> in preventing and treating illness. TCM practitioners

consider that food and medicine come from the same source, are based on the same basic theories, and have the same uses. Therefore along with the development of TCM many unique traditional Chinese functional foods were developed by combining food with food and food with herbal medicines.

He goes on to cite such examples as stewed chicken with ginseng for improving Qi (vital energy), stewed duck egg with green tea for diabetes, and fish head soup with gastrodia for hypertension. The influence of Eastern medicine including TCM on American food products can be seen in such products as menthol candy and rhubarb wine, which are used in Europe to improve digestion, and red yeast rice, which is used to lower cholesterol.

The documented use of functional foods in the history of traditional Chinese medicine began as early as 1000 B.C. in the West Zhou dynasty. The term medicinal food—food used for medical purposes—was frequently found in the literature of the East Han dynasty in 100 B.C., and another quite similar term— Fa Shan, or special foods—was used in medical works in the Song dynasty in 1000 A.D. The TCM theories and applied knowledge of food and nutrition were described extensively in most classical TCM publications such as *Yellow Emperor's Internal Classics* (745-221 B.C.), *Treatise on Febrile Diseases* (210 A.D.), *Synopsis of Prescriptions Worth Thousand Gold* (650 A.D.), and *Compendium of Materia Medica* (1578 A.D.) in which hundreds of functional foods and corresponding recipes were documented. In a medical work written about 1,400 years ago in the Tang dynasty, the use of congee make from rice husk or brown rice to treat and prevent beriberi and pork liver to treat nyctalopia (night blindness) was documented. Fe Hong's *Handbook of Prescriptions for Emergencies*, composed in 340 A.D. in the Jin dynasty, describes the use of kelp in the prevention and treatment of goiter and of pork pancreas to treat diabetes.

During the past 2,000 years, traditional Chinese medicine and pharmacology has spread to many countries becoming an important part of world medicine. Today the concept that foods have both a preventative and therapeutic effect is being increasingly recognized all over the globe.

RED YEAST RICE

Many Chinese suffer from atherosclerosis. In the United States, the most commonly prescribed drugs for this disorder are the HMG-CoA reductase inhibitors or the "statins," which include lovastatin, simvastatin, and pravastatin. The statins inhibit the enzyme necessary for cholesterol synthesis: HMG-CoA reductase. We will discuss how the HMG-CoA reductase inhibitors work later in Chapter 5. For now, let's just say that they are very effective in reducing cholesterol levels and are relatively free of side effects. However, they are also expensive and have limited availability to the majority of the Chinese population. This prompted Chinese medical investigators to search for alternative agents to lower serum lipids. Naturally they turned to traditional Chinese medicine for an answer. The ancient Chinese pharmacopoeia *Ben Cao Gan Mu* (Compendium of Materia Medica) recommends the use of red yeast rice to promote the health of the cardiovascular system.

TERMINOLOGY

Before we begin our discussion of red yeast rice, let's get acquainted with a few terms. Red yeast rice is a combination of two ingredients—yeast and rice. Yeasts are a group of 160 or so species of single-celled microscopic fungi. Not all are used in food production. Some yeasts are responsible for the spoilage of fruit and vegetables and others cause disease—for example, the common candida infections. Yeast has been used in food production for over 6,000 years mainly to produce raised breads and fermented beverages such as beer, wines, and spirits. The other component of red yeast rice is, of course, premium white nonglutinous rice.

According to Dr. Joseph Chang, vice president of Pharmanex and one of the authors of several studies on red yeast rice, "Yeast has always been popular and well-known in old Chinese technology. It is used to make rice wine and from there through trial and error they probably discovered or isolated a strain that provides this reddish color. The primary purpose of using this yeast strain was for the red color. The red pigment that is generated from the fermentation process comes from the red yeast and it infuses the cooked rice grain with this color. The red color doesn't come from the rice, the rice is just a nutrient for the yeast to grow upon during the fermentation process."

The type of yeast used to make red yeast rice is a species called *Monascus purpureus Went*. In Chinese it is called *Hung Qu* or *Hung-chu*. Red yeast rice can be milled to produce red yeast rice powder, also called *Zhi Tai*, or alcohol can be used to produce an extract of the powder, red yeast rice extract, also called *Xue Zhi Kang*. The red yeast rice research done in America used red yeast rice powder while that performed in China used both powder and extracts of various strengths. Both types are available for sale in the United States and appear to be equally effective. *Monascus* is also known under the name Angkak or as red fermented rice, red rice, or Koji.

When the term "red yeast rice" is mentioned in this book, it refers to the strain of *Monascus purpureus Went* that produces HMG-CoA reductase inhibitors. Just be aware that not all strains of red yeast rice contain these active ingredients so not all foods or supplements that contain red yeast rice are going to be equally effective in lowering cholesterol. That is why you must purchase your supplements from a reliable source.

The active ingredients in red yeast rice are called mona-colins, and the chief monacolin is *monacolin K* or *mevinolin*. The chemical name that was assigned to this molecule by the U.S. Drug Nomenclature Agency is *lovastatin,* and the brand name of lovastatin made by Merck is *Mevacor*. All you need to remember is that monacolin K, mevinolin, lovastatin, and Mevacor all refer to the same molecule. The only difference is how it comes packaged.

CULINARY USE OF RED YEAST RICE

Red yeast rice is a relative of the yellow yeast rice that is also used in traditional Chinese medicine and to produce miso. Red yeast rice is a dietary staple in many Asian countries. Since ancient times it has been used in China, Taiwan, and Okinawa to brew alcoholic beverages and contribute color, flavor, and aroma to food. Traditionally it is grown on white rice and then both the growing yeast and the rice is ground up to produce a condiment. It has been used as a food preservative to maintain the color and taste of fish and meat and as a flavoring and col-oring agent in a number of traditional Chinese foods. Red yeast rice is what puts the red into Peking duck. Dr. Chang explained, "It's very spicy in general not like chili pepper spicy but just has a spicy flavor to it. Traditionally it has been used as a part of a condiment to flavor roast duck. When you go into Chinatown you see a lot of restaurants with roast ducks hanging in the window. Traditionally the recipe calls for red yeast rice to give it that red tint you find on roast duck or pork so it is used in that way as a food flavoring agent."

It is also used to make rice wine. According to Dr Chang, "Red yeast rice is used to make rice wine. When a girl was born in a particular northern province in China it has always been the custom of the girl's family to immediately start making rice wine with red yeast. And the way they do it is this. They do the fermentation process and bury all the jars in the back yard—it's very cold in the northern provinces—and that's where it will stay and continue the fermentation process until the girl reaches marriageable age about 13 or 14. And then on the day of the marriage these jars of wine are retrieved from the ground and used as part of the dowry for the girl to the husband or to the husband's family. It is highly prized."

Although red yeast rice had its beginnings in China it is also a dietary staple in Japan and other Asian countries. The earliest reported attempt to manufacture red yeast rice in the United States was in 1920 by Margaret B. Church, an employee of the Bureau of Chemistry, U.S. Department of Agriculture, the direct predecessor to the Food and Drug Administration. Red yeast rice has been used in the Asian-American community in the United States since World War II.

Red yeast rice is also used in Europe where *Monascus* became known by the description of Netherlands scientists, who isolated and classified various *Monascus* species from the red yeast used in Java. In Europe there is a strong interest in using red yeast rice as an agent to color food. The Institute of Meat Research in Kulmbach, Germany, has proposed that red yeast rice be substituted for the nitrite-curing salts commonly used today to preserve the red color of meat in hot dogs, bacon, sausage, and other processed meat products. Although they make the product look nice and fresh, nitrites may be dangerous to your health. If eaten, they form compounds in the stomach called nitrosamines, which cause cancer in animals and are strongly linked to stomach cancers in humans. When red yeast rice is used in meat and meat products, they gain a more intense red hue that is very stable under great heat, light, oxygen, and pH changes. The red pigments found in *Monascus* are Monascorubin and Monascin.

MEDICINAL USE OF
RED YEAST RICE

More important to us here are the health effects of red yeast rice. For over two thousand years, the medicinal effects of this food have been known and used in China. The first use of red yeast rice was documented in the T'ang dynasty in 800 A.D., and it has been used since then as a food additive and medicinal agent. *Monascus* was also mentioned for producing "brewed alcoholic drinks" (Arrack) in 1331 in "Yin Shan Zhang Yao." Instructions on how to make red yeast rice can be found in an ancient Chinese treatise on herbs, the monograph of Li Shih-Chun *Compendium of Materia Medica* (*Ben Cao Gang Mu*-Dan Shi Bu Yi) published during the Ming dynasty (1368-1644).

In this text, red yeast rice "sanctions the digestion, vitalizes the blood, strengthens the spleen and dries the stomach. You treat red and white dysentery [with it] and take it with fixed and fluid food . . . Hongqu has the ability to cure stomach and spleen, to strengthen the blood, and the principle to preserve and endorse the common Qi interdependent." It is also mentioned as a component of several herbal preparations for the treatment of indigestion, diarrhea, and heart and abdominal pains.

The prototype HMG-CoA reductase inhibitor was mevastatin, which was discovered in extracts of the fuzzy mold *Penicillium citrinum* by Professor Akira Endo in Japan. Because preliminary study suggested it may be toxic in animals, it was never developed for use humans. In 1979, Endo discovered another HMG-CoA reductase inhibitor—this time from a strain of *Monascus purpureus*. Endo named this substance monacolin K—also known as mevinolin and lovastatin. Today Merck's brand of lovastatin—Mevacor—is isolated from a strain of *Aspergillus terreus*, a mold.

PRODUCTION PROCESS

According to Dr. Chang, the production of red yeast rice has changed little over the years. "Some of the earliest lithograph engravings that we have from China dating back to the 17th century show that the rice is first cooked. Then the cooked rice is taken to the stream or fresh water supply and washed several times. The water is discarded and the cooked rice is then taken back and spread on bamboo trays. They sprinkle red yeast on top of the rice beds that have been created on the trays and then they allow the beds to ferment. As soon as the whole bed of rice becomes red that is the end of the fermentation process. They take it, heat it up to kill the yeast, and then pulverize or mill the rice grains into fine powder for use as a condiment."

How does that differ from how red yeast rice is made today? Not much, the process is basically the same. Dr. Chang explained how his company's brand of red yeast rice (Cholestin) is made. "Instead of bamboo trays we have a large factory of our own and have replaced the bamboo trays with steel sterilized trays. The other steps are the same. After the fermentation process we heat sterilize the red yeast rice to kill the yeast and then take it through a few more proprietary extraction steps to make it cleaner and get rid of any microbes and other contaminants. Then we do a second heat sterilization step which relates to the precise temperature that the fermentation is occurring."

The Method for the Production of Hong Qu (Red Yeast Rice), from Compendium of Materia Medica,1590

You take 1 Dan and 5 Dou Jing Mi (a special sort of rice). Clean this with water in a bowl and let it soak for one night. Then you'll cook it like normal food. Further you separate into 15 portions and add 3 Jin Pilzmutter. Roll and knead to distribute all equally. Form together to one portion and cover it carefully with a silk cloth. First heat, then take off the silk and splay. If the rice pulp is warm, push it together to a heap. Again cover it carefully. Next day at noon again make three heaps, let it rest for a while and form of each part five heaps. Let it rest short time. Then form all together to a heap. Then let it

The red pigments that made red yeast rice valuable for culinary reasons also make it valuable for medicinal reasons. According to Dr Chang, "Now we know that the chemical that goes to make up this red pigment shares the same similarities as the monacolins. So the yeast can go either way, in fact, it goes both ways. During the fermentation process it will make these red pigments and it will also make these more biologically active ingredients."

Sometimes an additional step is added and an extract is made. Alcohol is mixed with the red yeast rice powder. The colored liquid is poured off and allowed to evaporate, leaving crisp purple-red granules that are further ground into a powder. This extract takes up less volume than whole red yeast rice powder and allows the manufacturer to put more active ingredients into fewer capsules.

CHOOSE YOUR SUPPLEMENT CAREFULLY

This is why I cannot warn you often enough to chose your red yeast rice supplements carefully. Not all extracts (or whole powders) are equal. Not all strains of *Monascus purpureus* produce the same levels of active ingredients. Some produce none at all and so will not lower your cholesterol. There is also a fear among some manufactures that red yeast rice powder might be spiked with lovastatin by unscrupulous makers to make it more powerful.

rest for a while. Then form 15 pieces. Heat a little and then form again a heap. Repeat this 5 times. At the third day fill a big tub with fresh water. Dip short time and process wet and form again a heap. Handle again with this method. At the fourth day again dip it in fresh water. If the fungus falls for half and swims for half at the surface, then again use the method from above: Dip shortly. If the fungus completely is at the surface, it's ready. Take it out and dry it in the sun. If this rice responds, we call it sheng huang, a fresh yellow color. If you add Hong Qu to alcohol, fish sauces or hacked meat, it results in a fresh and appealing red. If it doesn't appease the heart, it's quality isn't very well. If added to medicaments, take stored, old Hong Qu, that's good.

The companies that market red yeast rice do not make their own product. They purchase it in bulk from suppliers in the United States, China, Taiwan, or Japan and then place it in capsules. The quality of the product therefore depends on the quality of the supplier. All of the companies I talked with had strict quality controls and always sought to purchase the highest quality red yeast rice. However, there are a few companies that buy only the cheapest to keep prices down and beat the competition. They do not care if their product works, only how much profit can be made. Because it so easy and cheap to market products on the Internet, be very careful when ordering supplements this way. Anyone can have an attractive Web site.

For this reason you might want to stick to the established standardized brands with good quality controls that test their raw materials. Do not always assume that the cheapest brand is the best buy. If your cholesterol does not decrease after two months of daily treatment, it may be due to the brand of red yeast rice you have purchased rather than an inability of the red yeast rice itself to work. Try again using a major standardized brand such as Cholestin before giving up. Remember, if your red yeast rice supplement is too good a deal, it's probably a steal!

HMG-COA REDUCTASE INHIBITORS

Which compounds in red yeast rice are responsible for its cholesterol lowering actions? According to James Rippe, associate professor of medicine at Tufts University School of Medicine in Boston, "As a natural substance there are hundreds of potentially active ingredients in Cholestin that could have contributed to the cholesterol lowering. Cholestin contains a range of HMG-CoA reductase inhibitors that probably contribute to the effect."

Why not just season your food with red yeast rice? After all, many people in Asia eat between 14 and 55 g of red yeast rice every day as a food. They sprinkle it on top of tofu for breakfast.

However, there is no source of culinary red yeast rice available in the United States. Besides, you must consume red yeast rice daily on a regular schedule in order to benefit from it. According to Dr. Rippe: "Although red yeast fermented on rice is used to spice traditional Chinese food such as Peking duck and spareribs, this is not an efficient way to consume the substance. The capsule form of red yeast rice contains a more consistent amount of the active ingredients than the amount people in China obtain from these sources in their diet."

As we have mentioned, the active ingredients in red yeast rice are the HMG-CoA reductase inhibitors. Of the many strains of *Monascus purpureus*, only three produce HMG-CoA inhibitors when fermented under specific controlled conditions. But *Monascus purpureus Went* is not the only organism to produce these enzyme inhibitors. Animals fed a mixture of probiotic microorganisms including Bacillus, Lactobacillus, Clostridium, Saccharomyces and Candida showed reduced HMG-CoA reductase activity. Whole amaranth is also suspected of causing alterations in this enzyme. Ever eaten oyster mushrooms? These popular mushrooms—the second most widely consumed mushroom in the world—contain *four* times as much mevinolin as red yeast rice. This is not unusual when you consider that Mevacor—the lovastatin manufactured by Merck—is itself extracted from the mold *Aspergillus terreus*.

ATHEROSCLEROSIS

Now that we understand the history of red yeast rice and understand that food can help us with our cardiovascular health, let's take some time to understand the cardiovascular system. The next three chapters explain the process of atherosclerosis and how high cholesterol levels can damage your heart and arteries. We will return to our discussion of red yeast rice again in Chapter 5.

2

The Anatomy and Chemistry of Atherosclerosis

Before we can discuss the process of atherosclerosis and how a program of diet and red yeast rice can aid in its prevention, we need to understand the organs and structures affected by this disease. This chapter is a refresher course in the anatomy of your arteries and heart and the blood that flows through them. If you familiarize yourself now with these structures, you will understand the process of atherosclerosis better when we discuss it in the next chapter.

Much of what this chapter covers is taught today in high school health classes. However, when I was in high school, and probably when most of you were in high school, little about blood lipids was known. Read this chapter carefully so you understand the rationale behind the Red Yeast Rice Diet.

THE CARDIOVASCULAR SYSTEM

You could envision the cardiovascular system as a network of closed pipes. The blood leaves the heart and travels through the arteries to the capillaries and then back to the heart via the veins. It travels this large circle over and over (which is why it is called circulation).

But this idea of blood vessels as pipes does not illustrate its dynamic qualities. I like to think of the cardiovascular system as a living river flowing through a series of intelligent, interconnected canals. These canals pulse with the rhythm of the heart, contracting and dilating to direct blood flow and regulate blood pressure. They penetrate deeply into your body to touch each and every cell. Your survival depends on how well your cardiovascular system is able to carry out its duties.

The best way to understand the importance of the cardiovascular system is to experience it firsthand. Ready for a tour? Our journey begins and ends in the heart.

THE HEART

Blood cannot flow on its own; it relies on the heart to produce the force needed to propel it on its never-ending journey. The human heart is a hollow vessel of muscle, roughly the size of your clenched fist, and shaped like an upside-down pear. Each heartbeat pumps blood into two different blood systems. The right heart pumps blood through the pulmonary artery into the lungs, and the left heart pumps blood through the aorta and out to the organs and tissues of the body. The heart has to pump nine to ten tons of blood each day, a cupful at a time with each beat.

The heart supplies blood to the body, but it must also save some for itself. As you can see, tissues on the inside of the heart have direct access to nutrients. Muscle tissue on the outside of the heart must rely on the coronary arteries for oxygen and nourishment.

THE CORONARY ARTERIES

The coronary arteries are the first arteries that branch off the aorta. The front of the heart is fed by the left descending artery. The circumflex artery wraps around the left side and together with the right coronary artery feeds the back of the heart. These arteries are the most common site for atherosclerosis. Later in this chapter we will examine the process of atherosclerosis in depth. For now let us just say this disease can result in partial or complete blockage of these arteries.

When the blood flow through the coronary arteries decreases, the oxygen needs of the heart muscle cells cannot be met. The cells begin to suffocate, and this is felt as a type of chest pain called angina. The familiar nitroglycerine pill that is put under the tongue releases nitric oxide, which temporarily dilates the cardiac arteries, improving blood flow and therefore oxygen to cells. If a coronary artery becomes totally blocked, the muscle cells of the heart die. This is called a myocardial infarction (MI) or heart attack. Other common sites for blockage are the inner carotid arteries and the vertebral arteries, which feed blood to the brain. When these become blocked, the brain cells do not get enough blood to function. If this blockage is temporary, it is called a transient ischemic attack or TIA. Lack of oxygen beyond five minutes kills brain cells and is called a brain attack or stroke.

ARTERIAL SYSTEM

Let's take a closer look at the arterial wall. The artery we are in has three layers or coats. The very large arteries have all three coats.

- The outermost layer is called the *tunica adventitia* and it is most noticeable in the large arteries close to the heart.

White fibrous connective tissue gives this layer structure and protection so it can withstand high blood pressures.

- The middle layer is the *tunica media*, which is made entirely of muscle cells. These muscle fibers are connected to nerves from the autonomic (involuntary) nervous system. In larger arteries this coat has an extra layer of elastic fibers (called the inner elastic lamina) that separate it from the innermost layer. This coat is able to contract and dilate thanks to its elastic and muscle fibers. Constant contraction of this layer is responsible for high blood pressure.

- The innermost layer is called the *tunica intima* and it is where atherosclerosis begins. Closest to the center opening (lumen) of the blood vessel are the cells of the endothelium, a single layer of flattened cells. Underneath the endothelium is the subendothelial space, a thin band of extracellular material embedded with smooth muscle cells and white blood cells.

THE ENDOTHELIUM

We are standing now just outside the endothelium. Be careful where you step because this is the most fragile component of the cardiovascular system. It may look to be a simple lining, but in reality it is the brain of the cardiovascular system, so complex not all of its functions are yet understood. It regulates, controls, releases, converts, activates, and inactivates. The endothelium also manufactures a great number of messenger substances that "talk" to the circulating blood cells and the underlying smooth muscle cells of the artery walls.

It is here that the process of atherosclerosis begins as a lesion in the subendothelial space. The endothelium also plays a role in the oxidation of LDL (low density lipoprotein) particles. We will talk more about this later in the chapter.

Being just a single layer of cells, the endothelium is extremely delicate. When blood flows too fast or with too much force, endothelial cells can peel away from the artery, leaving the subendothelial space raw and open to invaders. Chemicals, bacteria, and free radicals are other sources of injury. Its fragility could be called the Achilles' heel of the cardiovascular system. When your endothelium is not healthy, the rest of your body suffers. This is why we have included nutrients that strengthen these cells in the Red Yeast Rice Diet.

BLOOD

To the naked eye, blood is little more than a sticky red substance that oozes from cuts. Our experience with it is very limited: most bleeding cuts seal themselves quickly and form scabs that heal without event. As a result we tend to ignore it. Let's imagine we have put a drop of your blood under a microscope. What do you see?

First of all you notice that blood is not red. The liquid (called plasma) is really a light straw color. Second, you see a large number of cells floating about. These are the red blood cells (erythrocytes), white blood cells (leukocytes), and platelets. All three cell types are affected by atherosclerosis.

The large cells you see are the leukocytes or white blood cells. They are part of the body's immune system. Unlike the other blood cells, which depend on the plasma to get them around, all leukocytes are motile. They are able to move themselves in and out of capillaries by squeezing in between the endothelial cells that form them. The white blood cells with granules are the neutrophils, eosinophils, and basophils, and the ones without granules are the lymphocytes and monocytes. In this book we will mainly be concerned with monocytes.

If you look carefully at our slide, you will see a monocyte "eating" another cell. One of the functions of this white cell is phagocytosis—the engulfment and digestion of bacteria, viruses, fungi, and other harmful-appearing particles. Later in this chapter we will see how monocytes stick to injured endothelial cells and slide under the lining into the subendothelial space. There they feed on oxidized cholesterol and morph into the foam cells that form atherosclerotic plaque.

Red blood cells are easy to recognize since they are . . . well . . . red. This red color comes from the iron-containing pigment, hemoglobin, the oxygen transport molecule. The hemoglobin picks up oxygen in the lungs to deposit later in far away tissues. Although they resemble Frisbees, they are pliable enough to pass through narrow capillaries and slide in between endothelial cells. The average adult has about 30 trillion of them, give or take a million.

The third cell type is the platelets. These are irregular spindle-shaped bodies smaller than the red blood cells. Platelets are difficult to recognize on our imaginary slide. As soon as blood is drawn they stick to each other and onto every surface with which they come into contact, sort of like two-sided tape. This ability to get sticky is how platelets stop blood flow and regulate blood clotting.

Researchers gave a group of thirty-eight healthy smokers either a single dose of 100–120 mg of Pycnogenol, a trademarked natural extract made from the bark of French maritime pine tree, or 500 mg of aspirin. They found that the Pycnogenol significantly reduced platelet aggregation, a condition that occurs when platelets stick together and form clumps in the blood. A clump of cells in an artery narrowed by atherosclerosis can produce a stroke or heart attack.

When you experience stress of any kind (even smoking), your body believes itself to be under attack and prepares for fight or flight by releasing large amounts of the stress hormone adrenaline. One of the affects of adrenaline is to cause the platelets that circulate in your bloodstream to aggregate or clump together. This ensures that any bleeding from any

Normally platelets move passively without interacting with endothelial cells or each other. When a blood vessel is cut, sticky molecules (glycoproteins) appear on the surface of the platelets and cling to the vessel wall to prevent blood loss. Sometimes the sticky response is set off when there is no injury, and platelets stick to each other, forming a clot. This can happen when the platelets encounter injured endothelial cells or the rough cap of a plaque lesion. The clot can then block narrowed arteries. You can help prevent heart or brain attacks by preventing platelet stickiness.

The straw-colored liquid in which all of these blood cells are floating is called blood plasma. Made mostly of water, plasma transports a wide variety of substances including compounds formed by metabolism (such as lactic acid, creatine, and uric acid), respiratory gases (oxygen and carbon dioxide), regulatory substances (including hormones, cytokines, and enzymes), nutrients (including amino acids, glucose, vitamins, and minerals), and of course the lipoproteins (including LDL, VLDL, and HDL).

Now that we have finished our little tour, we will take a closer look at some of these substances that are involved in atherosclerosis.

"wounds" gotten in the "fight" will stop bleeding faster and is one reason why heart attacks and stroke often happen during times of stress.

Participants were told to smoke (the stressor used to cause platelet aggregation) after taking the Pycnogenol or aspirin and two hours later had their blood drawn. The researchers found that a single, smaller dose of Pycnogenol was just as effective at preventing platelet aggregation as a five times larger dose of aspirin. This is good news for those who cannot tolerate aspirin because it increases bleeding and causes stomach problems.

Pycnogenol and pine bark extracts are sold as supplements in health food stores, pharmacies, and other retail outlets. They are also excellent antioxidants.

WHAT ARE LIPIDS?

When you think about cardiovascular disease, the very first substance you think of is fat. We have been told that fat is what causes atherosclerosis. Before we condemn this nutrients let's learn what it is and examine the evidence. You may be surprised.

Fat is another word for lipids. This diverse class of nutrients includes all carbon-containing substances that do not dissolve in water: fatty acids (the building blocks of fats), triglycerides or triacylglycerides (storage fat), phospholipids (phosphate-containing lipids), lipoproteins (protein-containing lipids), glycolipids (carbohydrate-containing lipids), sulpholipids (sulfur-containing lipids) and fat-related compounds such as the fat-soluble vitamins A, D, E, and K, coenzyme Q10, sterols such as cholesterol, and certain phytonutrients such as the carotenes. Many of the active compounds in red yeast rice belong to the lipid class.

WHAT ARE FATTY ACIDS?

Fatty acids are the building blocks of fats much like amino acids are the building blocks of protein. No food is composed of just one type of fatty acid; each has its own unique combination. It is this combination that determines an individual food's affect on your cardiovascular health.

The foundation of the fatty acid is a chain of carbon atoms. Since each carbon atom has four arms with which to bind (bond), adjacent carbon atoms can hold one (single), two (double), or three (triple) hands or bonds. If a carbon atom finds itself with a free hand, it quickly grabs onto one of the plentiful hydrogen atoms always available. At one end of the carbon chain there is a methyl group (one carbon with three hydrogen atoms attached). At the other end is a carboxyl group (one carbon with an oxygen and one oxygen with one hydrogen).

There are three types of fatty acids in the foods we eat: saturated, polyunsaturated, and monounsaturated. No food is made up of a single fatty acid; food contains different levels of two or three. For example, most people think butter contains only saturated fat. The fact is that almost one-third (32 percent) of its fatty acids are monounsaturated. The remaining fatty acids are saturated (65 percent) and polyunsaturated fatty acids (3 percent).

WHAT ARE POLYUNSATURATED FATTY ACIDS?

When adjacent carbons in a chain hold two hands (or have two bonds) between them instead of one, it is said to be a double bond. "Poly" means "many," so a polyunsaturated fatty acid is a fatty acid with many (two or more) double bonds. The polyunsaturated fatty acids (PUFAs) you eat are incorporated into the membranes of your cells and into the lipoprotein molecules that carry cholesterol.

It is easy to recognize PUFAs; at room temperature they are liquids. Their double bonds cause a kink in the molecule and this kink prevents the molecule from stacking straight. As a result, the PUFAs slip over themselves making them a liquid. PUFAs are found mainly in plant foods.

These double bonds are very attractive to oxygen molecules, which attack the double bonds, changing them into single bonds by adding an oxygen molecule. The result is an oxidized PUFA, one of the types of fat most strongly implicated in atherosclerosis. Other types of free radicals can also break double bonds. PUFAs can become oxidized outside of your body as the result of food preparation, inside your body as the result of free radicals, or inside the subendothelial space where an atherosclerotic lesion is developing.

Scientists have shown that the amount of oxidized fatty acids in the bloodstream correlates directly with the amount of oxidized fatty acids in the diet and that dietary oxidized fatty acid accelerate atherosclerosis in lab animals. This means that you can decrease your chances of getting heart disease by decreasing your intake of oxidized fats. To do this avoid PUFAs that have been exposed to high levels of heat such as cooking oil and the foods cooked in the oil.

WHAT ARE HYDROGENATION AND TRANS FATTY ACIDS?

The food industry has found a method of preventing oxidation of polyunsaturated fats so that they have a longer shelf life. This involves a process call hydrogenation where all the double bonds are broken and the fat is saturated with hydrogens. Sounds good, doesn't it? If oxidized fats are the cause atherosclerosis, then hydrogenation has got to be the answer. There are several catches, however. Besides converting the PUFAs to saturated fats, this process also destroys the essential fatty acids present in these oils (the essential fatty acids contain double bonds). Worse, hydrogenation also causes the formation of trans fatty acids—a molecular configuration that does not occur in nature. Trans fatty acids are notorious for increasing blood cholesterol levels. In my opinion they are one of the reasons for the increase in heart disease in this culture.

Avoid eating excessive amounts of PUFAs and eliminate the major sources of trans fatty acids and oxidized fatty acids completely. In the next chapter we will explain how you can do this.

WHAT ARE SATURATED FATTY ACIDS?

When all the carbon atoms in a fatty acid chain all hold single hands, it is called a saturated fatty acid. Saturated because all the free hands are saturated (or taken up) with hydrogens. Since saturated fats are straight molecules, they form solid fats at room temperature. We usually think of animal meat and products as sources of these fats, but some vegetable oils, namely the tropical oils, are also sources of saturated fats.

Saturated fatty acids have no double bonds that can be oxidized, so fats that contain high percentages of them are very stable and resistant to oxidation.

If saturated fats don't form oxidized fatty acids, then why do they have such a bad name? It's a matter of the company they keep. Foods rich in saturated fats are usually also rich in cholesterol. It is the cholesterol that can be oxidized. Saturated fats, for all their stability, are also still fats and as such are concentrated sources of energy. In other words, too much will make you fat, and obesity is another risk factor for heart disease.

Sources of saturated fatty acids include beef, beef fat, veal, lamb, pork, lard, poultry fat, butter, cream, milk, cheeses, and other dairy products made from whole milk. These foods also contain dietary cholesterol. Foods from plants that contain high amounts of saturated fatty acids include coconut oil, palm oil and palm kernel oil (often called tropical oils), and cocoa butter.

WHAT ARE MONOUNSATURATED FATTY ACIDS?

By now I'm sure you can guess that monounsaturated fatty acids (MUFAs) have only one double bond. They are more resistant to oxidation than PUFAs but are not as stable as saturated fats. The main fatty acid in this group is oleic acid, an omega-9 fatty acid. Olive oil is the richest source of oleic acid although smaller amounts are found in other oils such as almond and canola oil.

Researchers believe the low incidence of heart disease in the Mediterranean may be due to a high consumption of MUFAs throughout the region. Some studies have found that oleic acid has increased HDL levels. The jury is still out on their effectiveness in preventing heart disease, but since virgin olive oil is also rich in antioxidants, you should substitute some of these oils for PUFAs in your diet.

MUFAs have been shown to lower cholesterol in general and decrease the production of all lipoproteins.

WHAT ARE OMEGA-3 FATTY ACIDS?

PUFAs are further described by the location of their first double bonds. When the first double bond occurs at carbon three, its omega or "n" number is three. Oils rich in the omega-3 fatty acids are important to your cardiovascular health and are commonly found in fish and fish oil. The three dietary oils in this group are linolenic acid, eicosapentaenoic acid (EPA), and docosahexaenoic acid (DHA). Linolenic acid is an essential fatty acid that your body cannot manufacture.

Both EPA and DHA can be manufactured by the body, but sometimes the body may not produce all that it needs. EPA and DHA are the two oils that give fish their atherosclerosis fighting power. These oils are particularly valuable for those with high triglyceride levels. In one study, researchers found that fish oil lowered triglycerides by 34 percent, rivaling those achieved with Gemfibrozil, a commonly prescribed drug. Fish oils also lower blood pressure, which decreases the risk of cardiovascular disease.

Sometimes a slight rise in LDL levels has been seen with the high doses achieved with supplementation. This can be prevented by taking garlic along with the fish oil capsules. Researchers found that a group given fish oil supplements decreased TAGs but increased LDL. The other group, who was given garlic and fish oil, decreased total cholesterol, LDL, and triglyceride concentrations.

Fish oil has benefits similar to those seen with aspirin, including:

- modifies the tendency of platelets to clump
- enhances blood vessel dilation by increasing nitric oxide (DHA)
- promotes healing in injured endothelial cells
- minimizes inflammatory response to damage in the blood vessels

Fatty acids from fish oil are linked to reduced risk of heart attack, report researchers in Finland. In a study of 1,871 men in eastern Finland, high proportions of two omega-3 fatty acids found in fish oil were associated with reduced risk of heart attack. Scientists measured blood levels of the fatty acids DHA (docosahexaenoic acid) and DPA (docosapentaenoic acid) in the healthy men. During the twelve-year study there were 161 fatal or non-fatal heart attacks.

Men were divided into five groups based on their blood levels of DHA and DPA. Those with the highest proportion of DHA and DPA had a 44 percent lower risk of heart attack compared to those in the lowest fifth. Men in the highest fifth of DHA and DPA also had higher HDL "good" cholesterol, lower blood insulin levels, and less blood platelet "stickiness," the researchers found.

The omega-3 fatty acids are also precursors for prostaglandins, messenger molecules that enable the endothelial cells to "talk" to local tissues. The omega-3 fatty acids produce series 1 and 3 prostaglandins, which send "good" messages that tell your arteries to relax, reduce inflammation, and prevent blood clotting.

Although the omega-3 fats are polyunsaturated and prone to oxidation, they provide other healthy benefits that make them an important part of a heart healthy diet.

OMEGA-6 FATTY ACIDS

Oils with the first double bond at carbon six are called the omega-6 fatty acids. The dietary fats in this group include the other essential fatty acid linolenic acid as well as arachidonic acid (AA), and gamma linolenic acid (GLA). Both AA and GLA can be manufactured in the body from linolenic acid, but not everyone manufactures enough GLA. In the American diet we eat too much AA.

The omega-6 fatty acids are precursors to the series 2 prostaglandins. These send "bad" messages from your endothelial cells telling your arteries to constrict and encourage inflammation and blood clotting. In addition to this, omega-6 fatty acids are polyunsaturates and as such are prone to dangerous oxidation. Having these fatty acids as part of your membranes and LDL particles is like having ticking time bombs built into your cardiovascular system. When left unprotected by antioxidants, a fatty acid with three double bonds is oxidized eighty times as readily as a fatty acid with only one double bond!

The American diet rich in omega-6 fatty acids is one reason we have such high incidence of cardiovascular disease.

WHAT ARE TRIGLYCERIDES?

You are probably familiar with the term triglyceride—a value for it can be seen on your cholesterol test. There are several different names for this important substance; the old term is triglycerides and it was sometimes abbreviated to "tri." The new correct name is tri*acyl*glycerides, which is abbreviated TAG. In this book we will use a combination of the old and new: triglycerides and TAG.

Until now we have been talking about fatty acid, not fats. Triglycerides are the chemical form in which most fat exists in food and in the body. Its structure is simple: three fatty acids hung on a glycerol molecule. (See Figure 2-1.) After TAGs are absorbed by the cells in the intestine, they are packaged into chylomicrons—water-soluble particles—for shipment through the lymphatic system to the bloodstream. TAGs cannot travel through the blood alone since they will not mix with water. When they reach the liver, cells there package the TAGs inside other water-soluble particles—VLDL and LDL particles—for distribution to hungry cells throughout the body.

An excess of TAGs in the plasma is called hypertriacylglyceridemia, a condition linked to atherosclerosis. Elevated TAGs are often seen in people who have diabetes. Like cholesterol, increases in triglyceride levels can be detected by plasma measurements. These measurements should be made after an overnight fast. We will talk more about TAGs in the next chapter when we speak of lipoproteins. For now just remember that your TAGs are composed of the fatty acids you eat. If your diet is full of oxidized fatty acids, then your fats are going to be oxidized too.

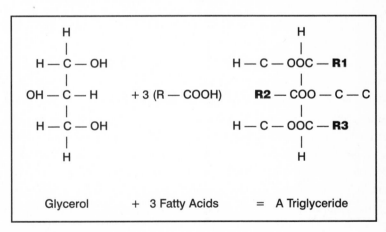

Figure 2-1. Triglycerides.
Almost all of the fat you eat is in the form of triglycerides. Triglycerides are also the form in which fat is transported in lipoproteins. "R – OOCH" stands for individual fatty acid groups. The properties of the individual fatty acids determine the properties of the triglyceride to which they belong.

PHOSPHOLIPIDS

A phospholipid is very similar in structure to a triglyceride, but it has one fatty acid replaced with a phosphate group. Since phosphates are water soluble, this simple addition makes the phospholipid more water soluble than a triglyceride.

When a phospholipid is put into a watery solution an amazing thing happens. The water-loving phosphate groups arrange themselves near the water while the fat-loving fatty acids tails congregate together. The result is a sphere. Phospholipids form the outer skin of a variety of structures. A single layer is the shell of the lipoproteins: chylomicrons and VLDL, LDL, and HDL particles. A double layer with the tails facing the tails forms the membrane of cells and the little organs (organelles) within cells.

CHOLESTEROL

We end this chapter with the most infamous lipid of all, cholesterol. For all the bad press cholesterol gets, it is still a necessary nutrient. Your cells could not survive without cholesterol, so adults are able to produce all that they need. Chemically, cholesterol is part of the sterol family and is used to make many essential substances including bile salts and the sex hormones. It is an integral part of all body membranes, including the skin, and is also used to make myelin, a substance that forms the protective sheath around nerve cells. In the presence of light, cholesterol converts into vitamin D. Since cholesterol is fat soluble, it must be packaged in lipoprotein molecules for transport in the blood.

The cholesterol test your doctor performs measures the amount of cholesterol in the HDL and LDL lipoproteins. This is the cholesterol manufactured by your body. The other type is dietary cholesterol found in your diet.

If cholesterol is so important, how did it get such a bad reputation? It was noticed that in parts of the world where serum cholesterol levels are low, atherosclerosis is almost unknown. Decades ago it was suggested that lowering cholesterol levels might be a major way of decreasing risk of heart disease. This generated much research and the now well-established theory that lowering serum cholesterol decreases the risk of developing heart disease and other manifestations of atherosclerosis. For years this was misinterpreted to mean that lowering *dietary* cholesterol would also decrease the risk of developing atherosclerosis. This has been shown not to be true. In fact, most people can eat all the cholesterol they want without an increase in their serum cholesterol.

OXIDIZED CHOLESTEROL

Now some researchers are questioning if serum cholesterol is the true culprit. Cholesterol, being a fat, is prone to oxidation just like all fats, and recent research points to *oxidized* cholesterol as the risk factor. Oxidized cholesterol is found in processed foods high in cholesterol such as powdered egg yolks, ghee—a product created by heating butter to high temperatures—powdered cheese, and the products that contain these ingredients. Fast food is a particularly common source. Cholesterol can also be oxidized in the body by free radicals. We will talk more about oxidized cholesterol in the next chapter when we discuss oxidation.

PHYTOSTEROLS

Cholesterol is only found in animal fats. Plants produce their own kind of sterols called phytosterols. When eaten, these lipids appear to compete with cholesterol for absorption in the intestine, therefore decreasing the total amount of cholesterol absorbed. Red yeast rice contains several phytosterols including beta sitosterol, campesterol, stigmasterol, and sapogenin, which may contribute to its cholesterol-lowering ability.

Apart from its role in atherosclerosis, high serum cholesterol can contribute to cardiovascular disease by decreasing oxygen absorption. Recent research has found that a high cholesterol level in the surrounding plasma causes the membrane of red blood cells to become more dense. This makes it difficult for oxygen to pass through the membrane so red blood cells may not take on enough oxygen in the lung or deliver adequate amounts to the heart and other tissues. This lack of oxygen may be the cause of heart attacks and pain in the legs from peripheral vascular disease.

The message to take away from this is that dietary cholesterol is not bad for most people, but large amounts are not good. But then, too much of anything is seldom a good idea.

3

Lipoproteins and Atherosclerosis

Now we are ready to put the anatomy, chemistry, and nutrition we learned in the previous chapter together and discuss lipoprotein metabolism. This chapter is about the "alphabet words" used to discuss atherosclerosis and heart disease. You know, the words contained in conversations like this:

Doctor: Jim, I just got the results of your blood work back. LDL is high, HDL is low. I've seen you eat, so I know you have a lot of OxChol and mmLDL. And since you're an apple those TAGs have me worried.

Jim: HUH?

This chapter will tell your everything you need to know about your lipoproteins so you can intelligently follow your new diet.

LIPOPROTEINS

We talked a little about lipoproteins in the previous chapter. You will remember that they are a way of transporting insoluble substances through the blood stream. If fats were just dumped into your blood, they would form globules that would rise to the top of wherever the blood happened to be. Not a good way for nutrients to be transported. The body needs some way of making the fats dissolve into the blood. It does this by using lipoproteins.

In the intestine, carbohydrates are broken down into sugars, proteins are broken down into amino acids, and fats are broken down into free fatty acids and glycerol. A drawing of the structure of fat and its breakdown products can be found in Chapter 2 (Figure 2-1, page 31). Fiber, a type of carbohydrate that resists digestion, and other pieces of undigested food remain in the small intestine. Eventually they pass into the colon. The digested nutrients pass across the membrane of the intestinal villi.

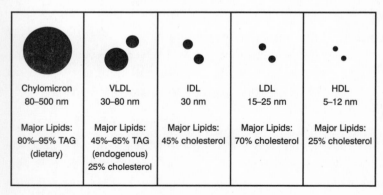

Figure 3-1. Characteristics of major plasma lipoproteins.

CHYLOMICRONS

The interior of an enterocyte (intestinal cell) is a very busy place. Some areas of the cell are involved in the manufacture of digestive enzymes and their shipment to the outside of the cell. Other areas prepare digested water-soluble nutrients and minerals for shipment into the blood. Still others must prepare fat-soluble nutrients for travel.

The cell uses some of the fatty acids to produce phospholipids, and the rest of the digested free fatty acids and monoglycerides are reassembled into triglycerides. Phospholipids are similar to triglycerides—but one of the fatty acids has been replaced with a phosphate group. As mentioned earlier, the phosphate group on the molecule is water-loving so the phosphate groups orient themselves to be closer to the water while the fatty acid part hides in the middle. When you put a group of phospholipids into water the "heads" of the molecule face out toward the water and the fat-loving fatty acid "tails" pull together. The result is a sphere.

This phospholipid shell is the basis for all the lipoprotein particles we will discuss. The water-loving outside allows it to move freely in the blood while the fat-loving inside allows it to contain a variety of fat-soluble substances. The large lipoprotein made by enterocytes are called chylomicrons. They are the largest of the lipoproteins.

That takes care of the "lipo" part of lipoprotein, but what about the protein part? Protein molecules are attached to the outside of the particle where they serve as identification tags. The protein found on chylomicrons is called apolipoprotein B-48, abbreviated apo B-48. When the chylomicron is ready to leave the cell, it must "show" this identification tag to the cell membrane in order to pass. Some people have a genetic defect that does not allow them to produce enough apo B-48. This means that chylomicrons cannot leave the cell and the enterocytes become engorged with fat. The name for this condition is type 1 familial hyperlipidemia or hyperchylomicronemia.

In simplest terms, hyperlipidemia is an elevation of lipids (fats) in the bloodstream. The five major families of plasma lipoproteins are:

- chylomicrons
- very low-density lipoproteins (VLDL)
- intermediate density lipoproteins (IDL) or VLDL remnants
- low-density lipoproteins (LDL)
- high-density lipoproteins (HDL)

Take a typical American meal that contains 30-50 grams of fat. The amount of circulating fat is 3 grams, therefore we would imagine that the meal would increase the circulating fat ten times. But it doesn't; circulating fat increases less than twofold. This is because when you eat fat it sets into motion a series of coordinated events that prevent dietary TAG from entering circulation while increasing TAG withdrawal.

The water-soluble components of the meal (including sugars, amino acids, minerals, and vitamins B and C) pass into the blood vessels that lead directly to the liver. The chylomicrons bypass this trip to the liver. Instead they enter the lymph vessels where they are carried in the lymphatic fluid up the torso and emptied into the left subclavian artery in the shoulder. During their journey in the blood stream they acquire more protein tags, apo C and apo E, which are donated by HDL particles.

The many chylomicrons from a rich meal will even make the plasma appear milky! They become a sort of "meals on wheels" particle, quickly seeking out the capillary beds with their millions and millions of hungry cells.

The cells use an enzyme—lipoprotein lipase—to unlock and distribute the triglycerides, phospholipids, and vitamins packaged in the chylomicrons. The cholesterol is unable to leave since none of the cells have the key to release it. It is not needed by most cells anyway, since they can manufacture their own when it is needed. After meals only adipose (fat storage cells) can access the TAG. Insulin released after a meal inhibits the lipase from other cells from releasing TAG.

This journey is complete within an hour when most of the chylomicrons finally find their way to the liver. They are much smaller but still full of all the cholesterol packed into them by the enterocyte. The liver cells are able to recognize the chylomicrons and pull them from the bloodstream. The sacs are digested and the cholesterol is finally freed. For now it is put into storage. All of this occurs very quickly, with half the chylomicrons being cleared from circulation in five minutes.

The empty chylomicrons or chylomicron remnants are believed to be atherogenic (contribute to atherosclerosis). How they do this is not yet known. The only way to decrease their quantity is to decrease the quantity of the fat absorbed in your intestine.

VLDL PARTICLES

In between meals, cells also get hungry, so the body has a mechanism for keeping food constantly available to them. It does this by sending out another "meals on wheels" particle, the very low-density lipoprotein or VLDL. From its name you can deduce that this particle must have more lipid in it than protein. VLDL particles resemble the chylomicron in organization but are much smaller in size. Its protein identification tag is called apo B-100, which is a single very large protein molecule.

The liver is able to manufacture a variety of VLDL particles in which density and size vary purely as a result of their TAG content. In healthy individuals with normal triglyceride levels, the liver produces a small VLDL particle. But as triglyceride levels increase, so does the VLDL size. Large VLDL are usually overproduced in those who are resistant to the hormone insulin (we will talk more about this in Chapter 9). This includes those who are overweight or who have non-insulin-dependent diabetes. These same groups also have large numbers of small, dense LDL.

The liver packs cholesterol into the sac along with the triglycerides and then releases them into the blood stream. The VLDL is carried to the capillary beds where it distributes triglycerides to hungry cells. As before, the cholesterol remains. Little by little the triglyceride is drained from the sac, causing it to get smaller and more dense.

Eventually, some of the VLDL particles find their way back to the liver where their identification tag is checked and they are removed. About half continue to circulate through the bloodstream, and these are now called intermediate density lipoproteins (IDL) or VLDL remnants. It is only twenty minutes from the time the VLDL particle was released from the liver to its return or transformation into IDL.

The IDL particles continue to distribute their triglycerides until they are emptied of triglycerides and only the cholesterol, phospholipid sac, and single large molecule of apo B-100 remain. This dense, small sac is now called a low density lipoprotein (LDL) particle.

VLDL ➠ IDL ➠ LDL

LDL PARTICLES

Now that the particle is empty of triglycerides, it starts to distribute its cholesterol. The LDL particles continue to circulate in the capillaries until they come into contact with an apo B-100 receptor. The receptor recognizes the protein and latches onto it so that the cell can pull the entire LDL sac inside. There it is digested and its parts used to make new cell components. If a cell does not need any more cholesterol, it reduces its production of LDL receptors so that fewer LDL particles are absorbed. The LDL that are not removed by cell receptors circulate in the bloodstream until they again reach the liver. Receptors in the liver recognize the particles and remove them. In the average person 70 to 85 percent of the LDL is removed by the liver with only 15 to 30 percent being removed by cells in the body.

As less LDL is absorbed by tissues, its concentration increases in the blood and more particles reach the liver to be removed by the apo B-100 receptors there. The liver recognizes that less cholesterol is needed and it decreases its manufacture. In this manner, the cells of the body are able to tell the liver how much cholesterol is needed.

A few paragraphs ago we mentioned that some people do not make enough apo B-100 tags. This allows a build-up of triglycerides in the intestinal cells. Without sufficient apo B-100, the liver also cannot remove LDL particles from circulation and will not recognize when to decrease cholesterol production. This means more LDL particles remain in circulation and the liver does not stop its production of VLDL containing cholesterol.

There are several variants of the LDL particle. LDL particles can become oxidized, producing a type called minimally modified LDL (mmLDL). We will discuss mmLDL later when we discuss oxidation. The second type is small dense LDL.

This smaller version is associated with high levels of TAGs and an inability of the body to use the hormone insulin. Treatments that reduce TAGs levels also increase LDL size. Small dense LDL is more easily oxidized than normal LDL and binds less easily to the LDL receptors responsible for removing LDL particles from the blood stream. This increases the time small dense LDL remains in circulation, perhaps giving it a more of an opportunity to interact and infiltrate the endothelial cells. The rate at which LDL particles cross the endothelium and enter the subendothelial space is related to their size. Small dense LDL will cross at a faster rate than either large LDL, IDL, or VLDL.

The third type is called Lp(a). Levels of Lp(a) over 300 milligrams per liter increase the chance of developing heart disease two-to five-fold. This type of LDL is due to a genetic variation that does not respond to dietary changes.

Nutrients that Prevent LDL Oxidation

- Vitamin E
- Vitamin C
- Vitamin B-6
- Carotenes
- Flavonoids
- Glutathione
- Coenzyme Q10
- Selenium

HDL LIPOPROTEINS

The last particle we will examine is the HDL or high-density lipoprotein. HDL is commonly referred to as the "good" or "happy" cholesterol since it is responsible for transporting excess cholesterol back to the liver for storage or elimination. About one-third to one-fourth of blood cholesterol is carried by HDL.

Medical experts think HDL tends to carry cholesterol away from the arteries and back to the liver, where it's passed from the body. Some experts believe HDL removes excess cholesterol from atherosclerotic plaques and thus slows their growth. HDL is known as "good" cholesterol because a high level of HDL seems to protect against heart attack. The opposite is also true: a low HDL level indicates a greater risk.

True to its name, HDL is the "leanest" of the lipoproteins as it contains the most protein and the least fat. HDL has two major apolipoproteins, apoA-I and apoA-II and five minor, apoC-I, apoC-II, apoC-III, apoD, and apoE, for a grand total of seven lipoproteins. When HDL leaves the liver it looks like a flat-round sack. As it collects cholesterol it plumps up and when filled looks like a ball.

HDL is the recycling truck of the lipoprotein world. It goes from cell to cell looking for excess cholesterol that can be returned to the liver so more will not have to be manufactured. The transfer of cholesterol is accomplished through cell receptors. Cells display an HDL receptor that HDL particles recognize and can latch onto. The contact between receptor and particle sends a chemical messenger to the interior of the cell, which returns with excess cholesterol. This is then fed into the flat HDL sack. As the sack distends it breaks contact with the receptor and the particle is free to leave.

But the particle doesn't always return to the liver immediately. When HDL particles come into contact with any lipoprotein containing apo B (the chylomicrons, IDL, and LDL), it can give them some of its cholesterol. This transfer requires the use of an enzyme called cholesterol ester transfer protein or CETP. Dietary fat is thought in some way to increase or decrease the activity of CETP.

When HDL levels are high, the risk of developing atherosclerosis is decreased. When CETP levels are high, the risk of developing atherosclerosis is increased.

HDL particles can vary in size among themselves. A research study done in Dallas in 1998 found that those with high levels of small HDL particles were three to four more likely to have heart disease than those with below average levels. This risk increased to fifteen-fold among men with both high small HDL and large VLDL.

HDL is thought to be responsible for ferrying cholesterol from various body tissues to the liver for reprocessing or elimination. In this way, HDL particles are thought to play a crucial role in reducing the risk of atherosclerotic cardiovascular disease.

WHAT IS ATHEROSCLEROSIS?

So now we know how cholesterol and triglycerides are transported around the body. Let's put it all together and see how the interaction between the lipoproteins and the cardiovascular system can result in atherosclerosis. I like to define atherosclerosis as an abnormal interaction between circulating oxidized lipids and blood vessel walls. It is a type of arteriosclerosis, which is the general term for hardening of the arteries. A certain amount of arteriosclerosis is normal as we grow older. Atherosclerosis is the major type of arteriosclerosis and the two words are often used interchangeably. It is a very slow developing disease. When you have been diagnosed, you have likely had it for many years.

What are your chances of developing atherosclerosis and heart disease? According to researchers leading the Framingham Heart Study:

- At age forty, the lifetime risk is one in two for men and one in three women
- By age seventy, the risk is one out of every three men and one out of every four women

According to the Centers for Disease Control and Prevention an estimated one million Americans will die from cardiovascular disease in 1998 and every year in the near future. I find these statistics rather frightening.

THE PROCESS OF ATHEROSCLEROSIS

Atherosclerosis is thought to begin with an injury to the lining of the artery. Monocytes from the circulating blood are also drawn to the injury and enter the subendothelial space where they are transformed into macrophages, white blood cells that eat debris. In laboratory tests vitamin E prevented the early stages of plaque formation by preventing these white blood cells from sticking to cells that line the artery wall.

Oxidized LDL (but rarely nonoxidized) particles penetrate the space. The oxidized LDL is especially tempting to macrophages that gorge on the cholesterol laden spheres until they swell, acquiring a bubbly appearance under the microscope. These are now called foam cells, and it is they who give plaque its bumpy appearance. The foam cells can hold only so many LDL particles before they begin to disintegrate, and the cholesterol forms a pool of lipid near the base of the lesion. The cholesterol crystallizes and, together with calcium, debris from dead cells, and collagen, forms a gruel-like, highly oxidized material (athero means gruel).

Smooth muscle cells from the middle muscular layer of the blood vessel migrate to this area as well. They multiply and secrete connective tissue proteins forming a connective tissue matrix or cap. As the plaque grows it presses into the middle layer compressing it and pushes into the lumen, decreasing the opening of the artery. The lesion is separated from the inside of the artery by a wall of collagen and smooth muscle called the cap of the plaque. Only the cap lies between the lesion and the blood. Heart attacks and strokes and other "acute" events take place when the cap ruptures. The lesion itself causes no symptoms.

The cap of a plaque lesion can be either stable or unstable. Stable plaque has a thick fibrous cover over a small lipid center. This type of plaque grows slowly, decreasing blood vessel size gradually. Unstable plaque has a thin fibrous cover over a large lipid center. This type easily cracks open, spilling the oxidized gruel into the blood stream, which immediately triggers a thrombus and heart or brain attack.

Researchers have recently found that the surface of the cap can become inflamed and that the inflammation can actually weaken it, making it more prone to rupture and thrombus formation.

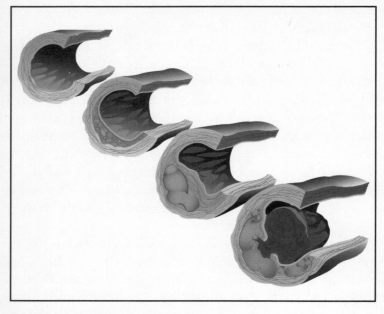

Figure 3-2. Plaque Development and Rupture.
Four phases of arterial thrombus formation include accumulation of lipid, fatty streak formation, development of a lipid pool and connective tissue cap and fissures leading to acute thrombus.

THROMBOSIS

A thrombus is a clotted mass of blood inside a blood vessel (erroneously referred to as a blood clot). It's formed through a complex interaction among platelets, the endothelium, and the coagulating elements of the plasma.

Thrombi are dangerous because they can form quickly and immediately stop blood flow to the heart or brain. A thrombus can also give rise to emboli by breaking apart into smaller fragments that are then thrown into the circulatory system. Emboli formed in the heart or legs frequently get caught in the smaller arteries of the lungs and brain where they block blood flow.

PREVENTION OF ATHEROSCLEROSIS

So far, all evidence seems to point to the oxidation of LDL cholesterol as the event that starts and continues atherosclerosis. But how does LDL become oxidized and is there anyway it can be prevented?

OXIDATION AND OXIDANTS

Oxidation is one of the most common chemical reactions. Oxidation means to *add* either an oxygen atom or a positive charge to a molecule or to *remove* a hydrogen atom or an electron. Reduction is the opposite of oxidation, that is the *removal* of an oxygen or positive charge or the *addition* of a hydrogen or electron. In most cases, the oxidation of one compound is paralleled by the reduction of another.

You have probably heard about free radicals. One way free radicals injure the body is by oxidizing lipids in the tissues (called peroxidation). This includes the fatty acids that form the cell membranes of the endothelium and those found in LDL particles. When a fatty acid is oxidized it changes in structure and no longer functions properly. This in turn alters the ability of the membrane to function and the cell can die.

The fact that lipid membranes can be damaged by peroxidation has been recognized for years. However, scientists have just recently begun to appreciate how lipoproteins can also suffer this same damage. It is now recognized that normal LDL does not play a role in atherosclerosis. It will not damage endothelial cells even when the person has very high levels.

The real culprit is the oxidized LDL that contains oxidized polyunsaturated fats and oxidized cholesterol. Oxidized LDL can start the process of atherosclerosis by injuring the membrane of the endothelial cell. LDL oxidized in the test tube and oxidized LDL isolated from human plasma is very toxic to endothelial cells, killing them within twenty-four hours in the test tube. Luckily, highly oxidized LDL is rapidly cleared from the body. Particles with less oxidation (also called minimally modified LDL or mmLDL) evade clearance and are able to stay around long enough to cause damage rather than death.

Oxidized LDL is also taken up uncontrollably by the receptors on macrophages that have been summoned by the injury, causing foam cell production. It can also further damage the surface of plaque making it less stable and more prone to rupture.

A number of reports shows that mmLDLs are present in the plasma of subjects with a history of heart disease or with diseases that place them at risk to heart disease, such as diabetes. The levels of modified LDL also change dramatically following myocardial infarction and appear to decrease when subjects take antioxidant supplements, most notably vitamin E.

Scientists have shown that the oxidized fats and cholesterol from the foods we eat are incorporated into our LDL particles. The fats and cholesterol in LDL particles can also be oxidized after the particle is manufactured. The easiest way to prevent atherosclerosis is to reduce your load of mmLDL by eating foods that are not oxidized, increasing your levels of antioxidants through diet and supplement, and to reduce the amount of oxidative prone fatty acids in the diet.

After spending only thirty minutes in a smoke-filled room, participants in a study had losses in their blood stores of antioxidants, including vitamin C. By depleting the body's stores of antioxidants, secondhand smoke contributes to the oxidation of cholesterol and lipids and therefore atherosclerosis.

Researchers at Helsinki University Hospital in Finland measured antioxidants in blood from ten healthy non-smoking men and women after they spent only thirty minutes in a room full of cigarette smoke. A test, called TRAP (total peroxyl radical trapping potential of serum), measured the

ANTIOXIDANTS

Your body prevents oxidation through antioxidants. Antioxidants do just what their name suggests—they work to prevent oxidation. They do this by "volunteering" to be oxidized first. The free radical takes what is offered by the antioxidant, and the reaction ends without any valuable lipids being destroyed.

Your body has two families of antioxidants: antioxidants that are obtained from the food you eat and antioxidant enzymes that are made by your body to neutralize the free radicals generated as a result of normal metabolism.

The two major antioxidants in lipoprotein metabolism are vitamins E and C. Vitamin E is a fat-soluble vitamin that is transported in your LDL particles. People who do not take a vitamin E supplement have an average of only three tocopherol (vitamin E) molecules in each LDL particle. After the vitamin has been oxidized by the free radical it becomes a vitamin E radical with no antioxidant properties. If you have sufficient vitamin C in your blood steam, it will change the vitamin E back to its usual antioxidant form. One of the main functions of vitamin C is to recycle "used" vitamin E. In this way, the same vitamin E molecules can be used over and over again to protect the lipids in their LDL particle. Without vitamin C, vitamin E can be used only once. Of course without vitamin E the cell membrane would be damaged or the LDL particle oxidized.

capacity of all blood antioxidants to rid the body of free radicals. Passive smoking caused a 31 percent drop in TRAP values.

Free radicals are found in tobacco smoke where they can combine with cholesterol in the blood to make oxidized cholesterol, the dangerous form associated with atherosclerosis. Researchers said that the free-radical stress by secondhand smoke may have a more prominent effect on a nonsmoker than an active smoker whose cardiovascular system has a more permanent (oxidant) imbalance.

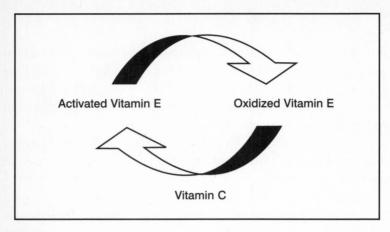

Activated Vitamin E   Oxidized Vitamin E

Vitamin C

Figure 3-3.

Other antioxidants that have been less studied for their role in heart disease are the fat-soluble orange pigment carotenes. This family includes beta and alpha carotene, lycopene, lutein, and cryptoxanthin.

Researchers at the University of Texas Southwestern Medical Center had already found that vitamin E supplements of 1,200 international units (IU) reduced plaque formation by 80 percent. In a new study they discovered another important effect of vitamin E on atherosclerosis formation: it blocks an enzyme that is a key to formation of plaque.

Vitamin E inhibits the activity of an enzyme called 5-lipoxygenase, which leads to plaque formation. The enzyme produces a substance that stimulates release of interleukin-1 beta, called IL-1beta, which promotes plaque in arteries. Earlier studies have shown that IL-1beta stimulates the adhesion of white blood cells to the lining of an artery promoting cholesterol in cells. Increased levels of IL-1beta have also been found in the coronary arteries of patients with heart disease.

Flavonoids are another large family of pigments with antioxidant activity. They include rutin, quercetin, myricetin, and the citrus flavones. Other pigments that neutralize free radicals are the proanthocyanidins, tannins, and anthocyanins.

ANTIOXIDANT ENZYMES

Although some vitamins, minerals, and phytochemicals act as antioxidants, the body's primary defense against free radicals is its enzyme system. These enzymes are manufactured by the body as long as it has all the raw materials it needs. The manufacture of these enzyme systems is under the control of your genes. Some people inherit strong systems and others weak. A strong enzyme system is what prevents some smokers from developing cancer.

Glutathione peroxidase is the antioxidant enzyme, used primarily by the cells of the liver, lungs, heart, and blood. Its job is to inactivate the hydrogen peroxide free radical and to search for lipid peroxides, the free radicals formed when oxygen radicals attack the unsaturated fatty acids of the cell membranes.

The mineral selenium is a cofactor of this enzyme and vitamins C and E enhance its effects. Glutathione and the amino acid cysteine can increase glutathione peroxidase levels. Both these nutrients are found in many foods, or you can obtain them as a supplement. You will find a list of glutathione-rich foods in Chapter 7.

The other two antioxidant enzymes are superoxide dismutase (SOD) and catalase. SOD prevents damage by the superoxide free radical. If not stopped, the superoxide free radical degenerates into the lethal hydroxyl radical that can steal electrons from virtually any organic molecule in the immediate area. When SOD works in the mitochondria it requires manganese, and when used in the cytoplasm it requires both copper and zinc.

Catalase is the enzyme that completes the reaction started by SOD by reducing the hydrogen peroxide radical formed by SOD to oxygen and water. It requires the mineral iron as a cofactor.

WHAT DOES ATHEROSCLEROSIS
DO TO THE BODY?

Although we tend to equate atherosclerosis with heart disease, it can effect any artery in the cardiovascular system. Most often however, atherosclerosis occurs in the heart, brain, kidneys, lower extremities, and small intestine. The good news is that lowering cholesterol levels with a program such as the Red Yeast Rice Diet can stop or even reverse atherosclerosis in all arteries.

ATHEROSCLEROSIS AND THE BRAIN

Unlike the heart, the brain needs a constant uninterrupted flow of blood with its life-giving oxygen. If blood flow through an artery is stopped, nerve cells served by that vessel die within three to four minutes. This interruption of blood flow is called a stroke or brain attack.

There are many similarities between brain attacks and heart attacks. The most common cause of both is atherosclerosis, which narrows the arteries with plaque lesions so that loose plaque or clotted blood can totally block an artery.

When blood flow is temporarily decreased a person can experience what is called a transient ischemic attack or TIA. The symptoms for TIA are the same as for a stroke, but they appear for a shorter period of time and then disappear. A TIA is a warning sign that something is wrong.

You don't have to rely on antioxidant pills to prevent oxidation. You can get them from food. Researchers at Johns Hopkins University in Baltimore studied 123 healthy people over eleven weeks to determine how diet affected lipid oxidation. During the first three weeks of the trial, study participants ate a control diet that was low in fruits, vegetables, and dairy products (defined as four servings of fruits and vegetables per day) with 37 percent of calories from fat.

After eating the control diet for three weeks, participants were randomly assigned to one of three diets, which they followed for eight weeks.

- One group of forty people continued on the control diet.

ATHEROSCLEROSIS AND IMPOTENCE

It is estimated that ten to twenty million Americans suffer from erectile dysfunction or impotence. Over 25 percent of Americans over fifty suffer from it.

In men over fifty, the most common cause of erectile dysfunction is atherosclerosis. Atherosclerosis in this instance occurs in the penile artery, the blood vessel that supplies blood to the artery during erection. This dysfunction can range from the total inability to gain an erection to a decrease in the strength of the erection. Erectile dysfunction is a warning that other more vital arteries may be blocked. In this instance, reversing atherosclerosis will not only save your life, it might even liven up your sex life!

ATHEROSCLEROSIS AND PERIPHERAL VASCULAR DISEASE (PVD)

Peripheral vascular disease (PVD) is a common disorder in the United States, affecting 8.4 million people. Of these, roughly 3.4 million experience a mild form of PVD called intermittent claudication, pain in the legs upon exercise. This pain is caused by a lack of oxygen to the muscle tissue, and the pain subsides within a few minutes of stopping the exercise. Atherosclerosis, which narrows the arteries that supply blood to the legs, decreases the amount of oxygen available. This amount is sufficient for the muscle cells when they are at rest, but when

- A second group of forty-two people ate a diet similar to the control diet with nine servings of fruits and vegetables per day and that was rich in potassium, magnesium, and fiber.
- A third group of forty-one people ate a combination diet with ten servings of fruits and vegetables a day, low-fat dairy products, and other reduced-fat foods.

Scientists found that those in the third group were better able to neutralize oxygen-free radicals and protect against oxidation of lipids. Blood lipids are altered, or oxidized, when exposed to oxygen-free radicals. Researchers said that diets rich in fruits and vegetables can increase the antioxidant capacity of blood, which protects against lipid oxidation.

exercised these tissues need more oxygen than the narrowed arteries can provide, and pain results. I like to think of intermittent claudication as "angina" of the legs. Like angina, it is a warning that something is wrong.

Recent research suggests that high serum cholesterol levels, apart from their role in promoting atherosclerosis, may decrease the ability of red blood cells to carry oxygen. It is this lack of oxygen that may be the cause of pain in PVD. Simply lowering cholesterol levels may bring immediate results as more oxygen is delivered to tissues.

An estimated 840,000 Americans have a more serious manifestation of PVD called leg ischemia, a critical shortage of oxygen in their legs. This oxygen starvation leads to muscle dysfunction and finally, if untreated, nerve damage, mitochondrial DNA injury, muscle atrophy, and gangrene.

ATHEROSCLEROSIS AND ALZHEIMER'S DISEASE

Atherosclerosis may be a risk factor for Alzheimer's disease, according to a new study. Patients with severe atherosclerosis were three times more likely than those without atherosclerosis to have Alzheimer's disease, according to epidemiologists at Erasmus University Medical School in Rotterdam, the Netherlands.

Researchers looked for evidence of atherosclerosis in 284 patients with dementia (207 of whom had Alzheimer's disease) and in 1,698 individuals without the condition. Dementia was 1.3 to 1.9 times more likely to develop in subjects with one of three indicators of atherosclerosis than in subjects with no signs of atherosclerosis, the researchers reported.

Patients with only one indicator of atherosclerosis were 1.3 to 1.8 times more likely to have Alzheimer's disease and 1.9 to 3.2 times more likely to have vascular dementia. Alzheimer's disease accounts for at least half of all cases of dementia. Vascular dementia previously has been linked to atherosclerosis.

4

Supplements to Use with
Red Yeast Rice

Red yeast rice is not the only food supplement that can lower cholesterol levels, although it is by far the most effective. You may want to try some of these others to help lower your cholesterol numbers even more. Since all of these supplements use different mechanisms to lower cholesterol, they can be used safely together with red yeast rice. All of these supplements also have other health benefits. They will help protect your body from various types of cancer and osteoporosis and aid your immune system in protecting you from infection. Many will also help to decrease other risk factors for cardiovascular disease such as high blood pressure and diabetes.

SOLUBLE FIBER

The benefits of fiber were first noted over thirty-five years ago by Dennis Burkitt, who noted that native Africans whose natural diets were very high in fiber had a very low incidence of certain diseases, including digestive diseases and diabetes as well as low cholesterol. The component of that high fiber diet that lowered cholesterol is soluble fiber. In fact, soluble fiber has an impact on all the major risk factors for cardiovascular disease. When you look at populations, a high fiber intake is associated with a decrease in total cholesterol, LDL cholesterol, and triglycerides, as well as lower blood pressure, improved insulin insensitivity, and diabetes and weight control.

Dietary fiber comes in two types: the kind that can dissolve in water—soluble—and the kind that can't dissolve in water—insoluble. Intensive nutrition intervention with diets rich in complex carbohydrates and water-soluble fiber have reduced serum cholesterol 20 to 32 percent and fasting serum triglycerides 10 to 20 percent. It accomplishes all this through several different mechanisms.

In Chapter 2 we learned that excess cholesterol is excreted as bile salts in the intestine, and ordinarily this cholesterol is reabsorbed. However, when soluble fiber is present, it binds the cholesterol so that it cannot be reabsorbed. The liver then must use its stored cholesterol to replenish the bile salts, and the total amount of cholesterol is decreased.

Although soluble fiber resists digestion by enzymes made by humans, it is readily digested by enzymes made by bacteria. The human colon (large intestine) is home to millions of helpful bacteria that feed upon the soluble fiber and then ferment them into gases, lactic acid, and short chain fatty acids (SCFAs). These SCFAs fuel the intestinal cells and help to prevent colon cancer. They are also absorbed into the bloodstream and travel to the liver where they influence lipoprotein metabolism in such a way that total cholesterol and LDL levels drop.

Soluble fiber also increases the amount of time food spends in the stomach and increases the time it takes for food to pass through the intestines. Because of this, sugar extracted from the food enters the bloodstream slowly causing a smaller increase in blood sugar and a correspondingly smaller increase in blood insulin levels. All of this is good news for those with insulin resistance. A high fiber intake significantly reduces insulin requirements of diabetic individuals by lowering plasma glucose levels. High fiber diets also have been shown to lower systolic blood pressure by 11 percent and diastolic pressure by 10 percent in people with hypertension. High fiber intake promotes weight loss and maintenance through increased satiety.

Because fiber has been shown to be so effective in lowering cholesterol, several companies now market fiber supplements. Of the many on the market, only two have done research on their products to back up their claims.

- Fiber Plan, from Shaklee Corporation, is a blend of four different soluble fibers: psyllium, pectin, guar gum, and locust bean gum. In two good studies, Fiber Plan lowered cholesterol. In the longer of the two, fifteen grams a day for six months lowered LDL by 14 percent in twenty-four men and women.
- Metamucil from Procter & Gamble is flavored psyllium seed. Six studies have looked at Metamucil's effect on cholesterol. Ten grams a day, one serving of three teaspoons, dropped total cholesterol by 4 to 15 percent and LDL cholesterol by 6 to 20 percent.

You can buy ground psyllium seed in your health food store. This tasteless powder dissolves easily in juice making a very palatable drink. A number of other natural laxatives also contain psyllium seed. Beware though, some fiber laxatives contain artificial fibers. They have a laxative effect but will do nothing for your cholesterol levels. Always read the label.

Oat bran and rice bran are also cheap fiber supplements— just sprinkle them on your morning breakfast cereal. The active component in oats is beta glucan, a soluble fiber, and oat bran is a very concentrated source of it. The active component in rice bran is not the bran at all but the oil. Rice bran is also a rich source of insoluble fiber. It is a good choice for those who are allergic or intolerant to wheat or oats.

The National Cancer Institute recommends that you consume 25 to 35 g of fiber each day, while the American Diabetes Association recommends 25 g for every 1,000 calories. According to the National Cancer Institute, the average American gets only 10 to 20 g a day. The Red Yeast Diet should increase your fiber intake substantially. Depending on your serving sizes it should provide you with 25 to 30 g of fiber. If your red yeast rice supplement does not lower your cholesterol levels as much as you need, you may want to consider a fiber supplement.

Fiber sources that decrease cholesterol

Food	Percentage Decrease in Total Cholesterol
Beans	16 percent
Oat and rice bran	13–19 percent
Psyllium supplements	13 percent
Pectin supplements	12 percent
Guar supplements	11 percent
Fruits and vegetables	7 percent
Soy fiber	6.6 percent

HORMONE REPLACEMENT THERAPY (FOR WOMEN)

After menopause, women have a greater chance of developing atherosclerosis. It doesn't matter if the menopause is natural, surgical, or premature, the results are the same—a loss of estrogen. Estrogen is believed to be the protective factor that prevents the development of atherosclerosis in women. The Postmenopausal Estrogen/Progestin Interventions (PEPI) trial looked at the effect hormone replacement therapy (HRT) had on CHD risk factors. Results from the PEPI study showed that:

- Estrogen-only therapy raised the level of HDL-cholesterol.
- Combined estrogen-progestin therapies also increased HDL levels, although less than estrogen alone.
- All the hormone regimens decreased the level of LDL cholesterol about the same.
- Fibrinogen levels were decreased by all the hormones, which may be a desirable change.
- None of the hormone regimens caused a significant weight gain.
- All the hormone regimens caused some rise in triglyceride levels.

However, many women do not want to take HRT because they fear they may get cancer. HRT has been linked to an increased risk of developing breast cancer. Other women want to avoid the weight gain that they perceive HRT to cause. This has led to a search for safer, effective alternatives. Soy protein is one such therapy that is very promising.

SOY PROTEIN

Epidemiologic studies that look at disease rates in different countries have associated low rates of cardiovascular, breast, and uterine cancer in Japanese women with a high intake of soy protein. An analysis of thirty-eight human studies found that when soy protein is substituted for animal protein, levels of total cholesterol, LDL cholesterol, and triglycerides are decreased. In these studies the amount of soy necessary for this effect was an average of 47 grams/day. However, favorable effects were seen with soy as low as 30 grams/day. You can get this amount of soy protein by drinking two cups of soy milk or eating a cup of soy-beans. We will discuss soy foods in detail later in Chapter 6.

Flavonoids are pigments found in a wide variety of plants that have beneficial effects on human health. Many flavonoids such as quercetin and rutin act as antioxidants and are associated with a decreased risk of cancer. Soy foods contain a unique type of flavonoid—the isoflavones—that are not found in any other plant. Isoflavones are phytoestrogens, plant chemicals with structures very similar to the mammalian estrogens used in hormone replacement therapy.

Foods such as flaxseed oil, dried seaweed, whole legumes, cereal bran, whole grain cereals, vegetables, and fruit are also sources of phytoestrogens. These foods contain precursors (the lignans) that can be changed into phytoestrogens (enterolactone and enterodiol) by gut bacteria. However, the isoflavones are the best-studied phytosterols. Research studies support the theory that the isoflavones found in soy protein may, like estrogen, protect against coronary heart disease. Estrogen and the phytoestrogens like isoflavones prevent heart disease by normalizing lipid levels.

Dr. Koudy Williams and colleagues of the Bowman Gray School of Medicine in Winston-Salem, North Carolina, studied the effects of estradiol (an HRT) and soy protein, given separately and together, on monkeys that had had their ovaries removed. All groups of monkeys were given a milk protein to produce atherosclerosis. The lipid profiles improved in all the treated monkeys. The researchers found a decrease in total cholesterol and an increase in the good HDL cholesterol in the estrogen-only group, the soy-only group, and the group that received both estrogen and soy. Estrogen and soy protein appear to work through different mechanisms to increase arterial dilation and decrease aortic cholesterol content. When given together, soy protein and estrogen may synergistically inhibit atherogenesis and improve coronary function.

Another study done at Wake Forest University Baptist Medical Center found that postmenopausal hormone replacement therapy markedly reduced the occurrence of atherosclerosis in the internal carotid artery in monkeys. Strokes usually occur because the internal carotid artery has become blocked due to atherosclerosis. This team found that HRT from soy protein with phytoestrogens provided equivalent stroke-prevention benefits to the standard Premarin therapy prepared from mammalian estrogens. In other words the soy phytoestrogens were just as robust as the Premarin.

The results showed that both forms of estrogen replacement therapy cut internal carotid artery atherosclerosis by more than half, compared to postmenopausal monkeys who did not receive estrogens. But neither treatment drastically reduced the size of the plaques. Both work best at preventing atherosclerosis from ever beginning. Once atherosclerosis begins to develop, both HRT and phytoestrogens have a small effect.

Soy protein contains a number of other atherosclerosis-fighting substances. Besides lignans it contains beta sitosterol—a phytosterol—and saponins.

The very best way to get soy isoflavones of course is to eat soy foods. There are a great variety of soy foods available—something to suit everyone's taste. However, if you steadfastly refuse to eat soy foods but still want the benefits of soy isoflavones, it is possible to obtain them in pill form. Look for a standardized isoflavone extract from a reputable supplement maker.

PHYTOSTEROLS

Just as plants have their own version of estrogen, they also have their own type of sterols—phytosterols. Phytosterols have a chemical structure that is very similar to cholesterol, so similar in fact that some cells in the human body cannot tell them apart.

Researchers have know for years that if you eat enough concentrated plant sterols with a meal, most of the cholesterol in that meal won't be absorbed. This is because the phytosterols and cholesterol must compete for the same absorption sites on cells. The more phytosterols there are to compete, the less likely cholesterol will "win" entrance.

To lower cholesterol levels significantly, you need at least 3,000 milligrams of phytosterols a day. The typical Western diet contains about 80 mg of phytosterols a day with campesterol, sitosterol, and stigmasterol the most common phytosterols consumed. Both a vegetarian and traditional Japanese diet contain only 400 mg a day. The only way you can use phytosterols for cholesterol reduction is to supplement them.

There are a number of phytosterol supplements available. These products can be expensive, however. Read the label directions carefully and make sure you are taking enough to be effective. Some of the supplements I have seen recommend lower doses than those used in studies. This makes the per month cost lower, but the results are not going to be as good. Recently, cholesterol-lowering margarines have started to appear in grocery stores around America. These products contain either sterol esters (derived from soybean and corn vegetable oils) or stanol esters (derived from wood pulp). Benecol, a Finnish margarine, contains sitostanol and in a study with 102 people lowered LDL cholesterol by 14 percent.

You can safely use any phytosterol with red yeast rice. In fact, red yeast rice contains several phytosterols although they are not in sufficient quantities to affect cholesterol levels.

GARLIC

Although garlic is a relative newcomer to the American medicine chest, it has been treasured for its medicinal value in Indian, Japanese, Chinese, and European cultures for thousands and thousands of years. It is perhaps the most useful of the functional foods. The more garlic is studied, the more fascinating it becomes. And studied it is. According to a report in the *Journal of the American Medical Association* the medicinal role of garlic has been the subject of over 1,000 scientific studies.

Hundreds of these studies have evaluated garlic's usefulness in treating cardiovascular diseases. Although dietary garlic has benefits, garlic supplements have been the most studied. Garlic supplements have been shown to:

- Decrease platelet aggregation
- Decrease platelet viscosity
- Decrease total cholesterol levels
- Decrease LDL cholesterol levels
- Increase fibrinolytic activity
- Increase HDL cholesterol
- Increase HDL/LDL ratio

One of the substances in garlic is a sulfur-containing compound called alliin. When garlic is crushed, cells are broken open and an enzyme is released that converts alliin to allicin. Allicin gives garlic its characteristic odor and is believed to be responsible for its antibacterial, antiplatelet, and lipid-lowering effects. The German preparations used in research are usually standardized for allicin content to imitate that found in fresh garlic.

Some manufacturers have developed an odorless preparation that allows the odiferous allicin to be produced in the intestine. The odorless alliin and an enzyme are dried and packaged in an enteric-coated tablet that protects the enzyme from destruction by stomach acid. Once in the intestine, enzyme and substrate are freed to interact, producing allicin and its conversion products. This way the yield of allicin is maximized and the problem of garlic breath eliminated.

Another type of product is aged garlic extract. Aged garlic contains S-allyl-cysteine, which is made out of allicin when the garlic is aged. In one study, researchers at Brown University School of Medicine found that supplementation with aged garlic extract lowered cholesterol levels and blood pressure in men with high cholesterol levels. Participants were forty-one men who had total cholesterol concentrations between 220-290 mg/dL at the start of the study. Half of the group was fed three aged garlic capsules (each with 800 mg extract) three times a day with meals for six months. The other half of the men were given a placebo. At the end of the six-month period the supplementation was changed so that the former garlic group was given the placebo and the placebo group was given the aged garlic extract for an additional period of four months. Low-density lipoprotein cholesterol was lowered by an average of 4.6 percent, and systolic blood pressure decreased 5.5 per cent with a smaller decrease in diastolic pressure. The researchers concluded that supplementation with aged garlic extract lowers total cholesterol levels by an average of 6 to 7 percent.

In addition to its lipid-lowering qualities, animal studies have shown that garlic directly affects the arterial wall by reducing the lipid content of the wall lining, preventing lipid accumulation that leads to plaque formation. In humans, regular use of garlic powder decreases the stiffness in the aorta caused by old age. Garlic is also a natural antibiotic, which will help stave off bacterial and viral infections, and it contains numerous anticancer compounds.

Not all garlic supplementation studies have shown a benefit. The type of garlic preparation used has varied from study to study including garlic oil, dried powders in the form of uncoated or enteric-coated pills, and aged garlic extracts. How the garlic is prepared affects its active ingredients, so if your garlic supplement does not work as well as it should, try a different brand.

FISH OIL

Back in the days when all fats were considered to be equally bad for the heart, a study was published that showed Greenland Inuits (Eskimos) had a very low incidence of heart attacks and diabetes. What was unusual was their very high intake of fat. Could it be that not all fats caused heart disease and athero-sclerosis? That high fat intake came from marine oils, and this study was but the first of many to show the heart-protective effects of fish oils.

As we saw in the last chapter, fish oil contains two very important fatty acids: EPA (eicosapentaenoic acid) and DHA (docosahexaenoic acid). When DHA and EPA are eaten, they partially replace the omega-6 fatty acids found in the cell membranes in practically all cells including the endothelial cells that line the arteries, red blood cells, white blood cells, monocytes, and platelets. When the cell membranes of all these cells are healthy, the interactions between these cells— which depend on healthy cell membranes—are also going to be normal.

Recent research has also shown that elevated triglycerides alone can be a powerful risk factor for atherosclerosis. One of the best ways to lower these elevated triglycerides is to sup-plement fish oil. Its ability to lower triglycerides rivals that of Gemfibrozil, one of the most commonly prescribed drugs for elevated triglycerides. However, three grams a day of these long chain highly unsaturated fatty acids can also raise LDL concentrations, especially in those who have high triglyc-erides. This is not unique to the omega-3 fatty acids, how-ever; Gemfibrozil does the same in similar patients. Just the same, many felt that this rise in LDL made the omega-3 fatty acids less useful. However, researchers at the University of Guelph found a way to prevent this rise in LDL while still achieving a drop in triglycerides.

Researchers there found that a combination of garlic and fish oil was highly effective in lowering the levels of total cholesterol, LDL cholesterol, and triglycerides. Their study involved fifty men with a cholesterol level greater than 200 mg/dL. The men were randomly allocated into four groups for the twelve-week long experiment. Group one took placebos; group two, garlic; group 3, fish oil; and group 4, garlic and fish oil. At the end of the twelve-week study period, significant reductions were observed for total cholesterol (12.2 percent), LDL cholesterol (9.5 percent), and triacylglycerol (34.3 percent) in the group taking both garlic and fish oil supplements. Garlic by itself did not lower triglyceride concentrations, while fish oils by themselves actually increased LDL concentrations significantly (by 8.5 percent).

The researchers concluded that supplementing with garlic pills and fish oils in combination is effective in lowering blood levels of total cholesterol, LDL cholesterol, and triglycerides while at the same time providing a beneficial decrease in the ratios of total cholesterol to HDL cholesterol and in LDL to HDL cholesterol.

All the other substances we have talked about so far protect the cardiovascular system by affecting lipoprotein metabolism. This does not appear to be the case for the omega-3 fatty acids. While they do lower triglycerides, their protective effect appears to be related to how they normalize the interaction between platelets and the blood vessel wall.

Omega-3 fatty acids differ from other fatty acids in that they are the raw materials out of which potent messenger molecules called eicosanoids are made. The eicosanoid messengers include prostaglandins, thromboxane, prostacyclin, and leukotrienes. They take part in blood clotting, inflammation, and muscle contraction and relaxation—all of which are involved in the development of atherosclerosis. This may be how omega-3 fatty acids protect against atherosclerosis.

The omega three fatty acids:

- Decrease thromboxane—thromboxane causes platelets to aggregate or form clumps. It also causes the arterial wall to constrict.
- Increase prostacyclin—prostacyclin prevents platelets from forming clumps. It also causes the arterial wall to dilate.
- Decrease leukotriene—leukotriene attracts white blood cells to the vessel wall.
- Decrease platelet-derived activating factor (PAF). PAF activates platelets.
- Decrease platelet-derived growth factor (PDGF). PDGF attracts macrophages and acts as a mitogen for smooth muscle cells.
- Decrease interleukin-1 (IL-1) and tumor necrosis factor. IL-1 and TNF stimulates smooth muscle proliferation and free radical formation.
- Increase endothelial-derived relaxation factor (EDRF)— EDRF reduces vasoconstriction and protects endothelial cells surface from blood clots.

They also decrease the thickness of the blood, decrease platelet stickiness, and increased platelet survival. Fish oil supplementation lowers blood pressure. Recent research has shown that supplementation with three grams of fish oil per day lowers blood pressure substantially in people with borderline hypertension. It also reduces how much arteries, which have been unblocked with angioplasty, will reclose (restenosis).

The combination of fish oil and lovastatin (one of the components of red yeast rice) was found to enhance the decreases in plasma triglycerides and factor VII. Elevation of the latter has been associated with a high risk of cardiovascular events such as heart attack and stroke. If you have high triglycerides, this indicates that fish oil and red yeast rice make a good combination.

5

Red Yeast Rice: Proof It Works

In the past few chapters we have talked about the history of red yeast rice, discussed the formation of lipoproteins, and learned how they cause atherosclerosis when present in high numbers. We have even learned about other supplements that can be used with red yeast rice to bring down your cholesterol. Now we have finally arrived at the meat of the book. In this chapter we will explore how red yeast rice works and discuss the research that proves it works. The rest of the book will lead you through the red yeast rice diet.

Just how much can red yeast rice lower cholesterol? In the American studies total cholesterol fell from an average of 254 mg/dL to 208 mg/dL in just eight weeks. In all studies the higher the cholesterol levels were at the start the better the supplement worked. Who should take red yeast rice? This supplement is not for everyone. Let's meet two very typical patients who illustrate who should take red yeast rice.

SUSAN'S STORY

Meet Susan, a young looking fifty-five-year-old. She looks the picture of health with her slim and muscular physique and active lifestyle. Although Susan was careful to see her gynecologist each year for a Pap smear and mammogram, she hadn't really thought it necessary to have her cholesterol levels checked. After all, atherosclerosis was a man's disease. She was very surprised then when a screening test at a local mall showed she was at risk for heart disease. "I always thought it was men who were over-weight and fat who got heart disease. I'm active and there is not one ounce of fat on me."

When her family doctor got her blood test results back, he recommended that she see a nutritionist. "Your LDL is too high although your HDL is fine," he told her. "But your triglycerides are also elevated. Before we try drugs, you need to clean up your diet." Her nutritionist explained how her junk food diet was part of the problem. "Even thin people can eat too much fat." The nutritionist recommended several supplements for Susan including an isoflavone supplement since Susan is post-menopausal, antioxidants to help protect her lipoproteins from oxidation, and of course, red yeast rice.

After four months of supplements, Susan's total cholesterol, LDL cholesterol, and triglycerides had decreased to acceptable levels. She has now decided to make a cholesterol test part of her yearly physical.

Susan is typical of a lot of older women. They fear breast and uterine cancer but forget that heart disease is the greater killer of postmenopausal women. In fact, cardiovascular disease is the major cause of death among adult women in the United States, killing almost 500,000 women every year, more than the number of deaths caused by all cancers combined. If you are a woman, don't forget you have a heart, too! Susan also didn't realize that just because her high-fat diet did not cause obesity it didn't mean it wasn't hurting her body. Susan was eating a lot of oxidized cholesterol in the form of snacks and fast foods. She was also not eating enough fruit and vegetables to get the needed antioxidants to protect her LDL and other lipoproteins from oxidation. Both the diet and the red yeast rice supplement work together to keep Susan healthy. Now Susan is as healthy on the inside as she looks on the outside.

SEAN THE OSTRICH

Sean Harris knew he was in trouble. The tense fifty-year-old carpenter had just had his first physical in years, and he knew before the doctor told him that his cholesterol levels were not good. After all, heart disease was not new to Sean's family. His father had died of a heart attack soon after retirement, and like his father, Sean had played as hard as he had worked. Both drank too much and liked to eat what they wanted, when they wanted, and how much they wanted. Both were overweight. Sean felt allright. He never had any chest pain or shortness of breath so he avoided having his cholesterol levels checked. His motto was if it isn't broken, don't fix it. But he could see he was following in his father's footsteps.

Sean was relieved to learn that his heart wasn't broken yet, but it was well on its way if he ignored it any longer. His total cholesterol levels were 245 mg/dL and his HDL was a very low 30. While his LDL was not high enough for drug therapy, it was high enough to convince Sean he was about to follow in his father's footsteps. His doctor put Sean on a Step I diet. Sean had already started to cut back on fatty foods and alcohol at the request of his wife, so it was not too difficult to follow.

When Sean returned six months later, the doctor could see that Sean had followed his advice. Sean was twenty pounds slimmer and had started a regular exercise regime. This was reflected in his HDL levels, which had risen by 7 points. However, his LDL levels had only dropped by 5 mg/dL. Sean was discouraged. "Isn't there some kind of drug I can take?" he asked his physician. The answer was no, his cholesterol levels were not high enough to start drugs. Then his doctor told him about red yeast rice and how it naturally contained the drug he wanted to try. So Sean started on a red yeast rice supplement, taking four of the reddish capsules a day with meals. He continued with his diet and exercise program.

Six months later Sean was back for another blood test. This time he wasn't disappointed; his cholesterol levels were significantly lower. His total cholesterol had dropped from 245 to 190 and his HDL has risen for 37 to 45. Sean now stands a much better chance of living long enough to enjoy a happy and healthy retirement.

HEALTHY ON THE OUTSIDE, SICK ON THE INSIDE

Most people with atherosclerosis do not look or feel sick. Many are like Susan—a veritable picture of good health—on the outside, that is. On the inside their arteries are choked with plaque lesions just waiting to rupture. Remember, for many men and women the very first symptom of cardiovascular disease is a heart attack or stroke. Forget the miracles you see on TV—one-quarter of those first heart attack victims die before ever reaching a hospital—that's over 200,000 people each year in the United States alone.

I know many men who are like Sean. I call them health ostriches. They put their heads in the sand and ignore all their risk factors because they feel fine. If your head is in the sand you know what part of your body we are looking at! Know your risk factors and respect them. Do the risk factor analysis found in

Chapter 8 and let your physician know the results. Your number of risk factors will change how your doctor views your cholesterol level. A cholesterol level that is low for a person with no risk factors will be high for a person with three or more.

WHO SHOULD TAKE RED YEAST RICE

In general, red yeast rice is recommended for men and post-menopausal women with moderately elevated cholesterol—over 200 mg/dL but under 250 mg/dL. If your cholesterol is under or over this level and you feel treatment is necessary, see your physician for guidance. Total cholesterol over 250 mg/dL must be monitored on a regular basis by a health professional regardless of the type of treatment the patient is on.

WHO SHOULDN'T TAKE
RED YEAST RICE

While red yeast rice is a safe supplement, there are certain people who should not take it. The growing body needs cholesterol or the brain and nerves will not develop properly. Therefore, do not take red yeast rice if you are pregnant, nursing, or may become pregnant, and do not give the supplement to infants, children, or adolescents.

Red yeast rice affects the metabolism of the liver so do not take this supplement if you have liver disease, are at risk of liver disease, or have a history of liver disease. Also do not take it if you drink more than two drinks a day (see Chapter 7 for the definition of one drink).

Do not take a red yeast rice supplement if you have a serious infection, disease, or physical disorder or if you have recently had major surgery or a major physical trauma. Do not take if you have had an organ transplant of any kind.

A PERSONAL STORY

For a testimonial we need look no further than Dr. James Eitner, a Board Certified Osteopathic Family Physician who works for Maricopa County Public Health. Dr. Eitner recommends red yeast rice to his patients with elevated cholesterol. "I recommend it for my patients with a total cholesterol of 200-240 mg/dL, or sometimes lower if there is a strong family history of cholesterol-related heart disease."

Dr. Eitner knows red yeast rice works because he takes it himself. Dr. Eitner had a family history of heart disease and his cholesterol levels started to rise when he turned thirty-seven. "It stayed in the 200–240 mg/dL range until I was forty, then jumped to the 280s." He tried several natural products, including a fiber supplement that decreased his LDL levels by 10 percent. However, that was not enough.

Dr. Eitner's insurance company was typical in that it would not cover the cost of drugs until his total cholesterol levels reached 250 mg/dL. One day Dr. Eitner saw Cholestin on a store shelf and decided to give it a try. He took the red yeast rice supplement for a year and his total cholesterol dropped to 160 mg/dL and HDL rose to 53 mg/dL. That's a drop of ninety points! Unfortunately for Dr. Eitner, Cholestin was taken off the shelves as the FDA banned Pharmanex from importing red yeast rice to fill its capsules. Dr. Eitner then turned to another brand he found at a health food store. This brand was using red yeast rice produced in the United States so they were not affected by the import ban on the foreign-made product.

Unfortunately for Dr. Eitner, this turned out to be one of those inferior types I have been warning you about. With the new supplement his cholesterol climbed to 280 mg/dL—a level high enough to qualify for drug therapy. His family doctor prescribed Lipitor, the brand name for one of the statins. Again, I'm going to caution anyone reading this book to make sure they take a quality supplement. As Dr. Eitner's experience shows, there are bogus supplements on store shelves today. With the Lipitor his cholesterol fell again, this time to a healthier 210 mg/dL with an HDL of 44 mg/dL. When Cholestin appeared on store shelves again after winning its battle with the FDA, Dr. Eitner added it to his cholesterol-lowering regime. After a few months his cholesterol level has fallen to 169 mg/dL and his HDL has risen to 52 mg/dL.

WHAT IS IN RED YEAST RICE

Being a natural product, red yeast rice is made up of many different substances—some of them active and some of them not. According to the research done on red yeast rice, it contains these compounds.

- Phytosterols—plant sterols that have a molecular structure similar to that of cholesterol; the sterols found in red yeast rice are beta sitosterol, campesterol, and stigmasterol
- Saponin and sapogenin
- Isoflavones and isoflavone glycosides
- Monounsaturated fatty acids including diene, triene, tetraene, and pentaene fatty acids
- Proteins, amino acids, saccharides
- Trace elements such as selenium and zinc

Although all of the above may contribute to the health-giving properties of red yeast rice, the active ingredients in red yeast rice are likely to be the HMG-CoA reductase inhibitors: monacolin K and its family of eight monacolin-related substances. According to Dr. Chang, vice president of research at Pharmanex, "As far as lowering of cholesterol, there is this family of monacolins and what we have identified as monacolins A to J. Particularly interesting is monacolin K, which also goes by the name of lovastatin or mevinolin, which was the original name. Sterols might contribute to it, but they probably play a very minor role in lowering cholesterol. There are other substances called fatty acids, both saturated and unsaturated fatty acids are present in red yeast rice and there is some scientific evidence particularly the unsaturated fatty acid may also help promote or regulate cholesterol levels in the body. That's as far as our research can tell us now."

According to Chinese researchers, "The mechanism by which M purpureus rice preparation reduces serum TG and raises HDL cholesterol is not completely understood. Decreased absorption of ingested lipids, reduced very-low-density-lipoprotein cholesterol are all events that may also contribute to a reduction in cholesterol and TG and an increase in HDL cholesterol."

In other words, even the researchers and manufacturers do not know for sure how red yeast rice works. This is not unusual for either herbal preparations or drugs. It is likely that the components with the greatest effects are the monacolins. Monacolin K or lovastatin is the monacolin present in the greatest concentration. A day's dose of red yeast rice—1.2 grams—contains 9.4 mg of monacolins. The red yeast rice capsules used in the Chinese studies had a monacolin concentration of 13.5 mg/day since they used a more concentrated red yeast rice extract.

The other components in red yeast rice may have other effects. I have heard claims that red yeast rice may benefit those with diabetes and hypertension. This may turn out to be true, but today there are no published studies or proof that red yeast rice does more than effect cholesterol levels. However, I wouldn't be surprised if red yeast rice had a few more tricks up it proverbial sleeve. This amazing supplement has just begun to be understood and more research is being planned.

HMG CO-A REDUCTASE

As mentioned earlier, cholesterol is an extremely important molecule that is used to make the cellular membranes, the steroid hormones, and bile salts. The word cholesterol comes from the Greek word "chole," which means bile. In addition to dietary cholesterol—that which is eaten in foods—a larger amount is made by the cells of the liver and to a lesser extent other tissues. This cholesterol that is manufactured in the body is the only cholesterol that circulates in the bloodstream as lipoproteins. Therefore, if you want to decrease the amount of cholesterol in lipoproteins you must decrease the amount of cholesterol made in the liver.

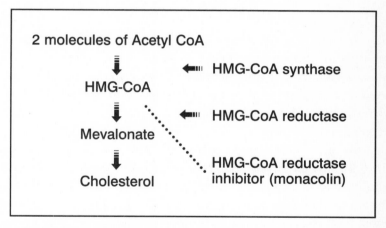

Figure 5-1. Two molecules of Acetyl CoA are turned into HMG-CoA with the help of the enzyme HMG-CoA synthase. HMG-CoA is then turned into mevalonate with the help of HMG-CoA reductase. If this enzyme is inhibited, less mevalonate, and therefore cholesterol, is produced.

Cholesterol is manufactured from two molecules of Acetyl CoA. This product is then changed by an enzyme called 3-hydroxy-3-methyglutaryl CoA synthase (HMG-CoA synthase for short) into HMG-CoA. This molecule in turn is changed by HMG-CoA reductase into mevalonate. The rate at which mevalonate is formed determines the rate at which cholesterol is formed. If less mevalonate is made, less cholesterol is made. The body makes use of this as a feedback mechanism. For example, eating cholesterol increases the amount of cholesterol in the body, which has the effect of inhibiting HMG-CoA reductase. Therefore, dietary cholesterol acts as a HMG-CoA reductase inhibitor. This sensitivity to dietary cholesterol varies greatly, as we are all aware. I can eat all the cholesterol I want with no increase in serum cholesterol. Others I know are not as lucky.

HOW HMG-COA REDUCTASE INHIBITORS WORK

If you wanted to find a drug that would decrease the amount of cholesterol the liver produced, it would be logical to find one that blocked the action of the HMG-CoA reductase enzyme. And that is just what the monacolins found in red yeast rice do. They inhibit HMG-CoA reductase and so are HMG-CoA reductase inhibitors.

But how does a lower cholesterol production rate translate into lower LDL levels? As production is decreased, the cells in the liver must find a way to get more cholesterol. They do this by increasing their manufacture of LDL receptors—the hooks used to grab LDL particles from the bloodstream—so there are more of them. With more receptors, more VLDL remnants get removed from circulation. Since VLDL remnants are the precursors to LDL, this increased clearance reduces the amount of LDL that circulates. Hence, the monacolins increase clearance of LDL and VLDL remnants.

RED YEAST RICE EFFECTS APOLIPOPROTEINS

In addition to its effects on the cholesterol feedback mechanism, red yeast rice extract has been shown to effect levels of apolipoprotein A (ApoA) and apolipoprotein B (ApoB). Studies done in China show that red yeast rice extract increases ApoA and decreases ApoB. You will remember from Chapter 3 that ApoA is found in HDL particles while ApoB is found in the LDL; therefore, a healthier lipid profile is one that has higher levels of ApoA and lower levels of ApoB. ApoA is also important because it is involved with the enzyme that frees cholesterol from blood vessel walls and tissue. This free cholesterol is then transported in the HDL particle back to the liver for disposal.

HISTORY OF THE STATINS

The first HMG-CoA reductase inhibitor was discovered in Japan in 1976 and named mevastatin. While Japanese investigators later showed that mevastatin greatly reduced serum cholesterol concentrations in men with hypercholesterolemia, it was never marketed because preliminary study suggested it may be toxic in animals. A related drug, lovastatin, was developed in the United States, isolated from a strain of *Aspergillus terreus*— a mold. Upwards of 10 million Americans are now thought to be on statins. Some experts say millions of people who aren't currently taking the pills should be.

They are the most commonly prescribed drugs for elevated LDL or elevated LDL with elevated triglycerides. They are also the most effective of the cholesterol-lowering drugs with a 20–40 percent decrease in LDL, 12–20 percent decrease in triglycerides, and a 5–10 percent increase in HDL. Side effects are mainly gastrointestinal and include intestinal gas, constipation, and abdominal cramps.

LOVASTATIN

Lovastatin is the generic name for Mevacor, a drug produced by the pharmaceutical company Merck. Mevacor is just one of five HMG-CoA reductase inhibitors sold today in the United States, the others being pravastatin, simvastatin, fluvastatin, and ator-vastatin. Lovastatin is produced by a strain of *Aspergillus terreus*, a fuzzy mold similar to the mold that grows on stale bread. Bacteria, yeasts, and molds produce hundreds of similar sub-stances, which apparently are designed to improve their chance of survival. Many of them appear as attractive or repellant fla-vors, smells, colors, or toxins.

The difference between the lovastatin in the red yeast rice and the lovastatin in Mevacor is that the monacolins in lovas-tatin are purified into crystals while the monacolins in red yeast rice are left in their natural state. Reputable companies will standardize their products—make sure that they contain the active ingredients they claim—but they will not cut the final product with rice powder or enhance it with purified lovastatin. The smallest lovastatin pill on the market is 10 mil-ligrams, while a daily four-pill regimen of Cholestin adds up to 5 milligrams of lovastatin.

SAFETY OF RED YEAST RICE

Red yeast rice and red yeast rice extracts have passed toxicology studies to determine if they were safe. These studies used much higher amounts of extracts than the typical daily dose for humans yet showed no toxicity.

In a chronic test—one that gives a very high single dose—24 grams/kilogram of body weight red yeast rice was fed to a group of rats. This is an amount equivalent to a 600 times the suggested dose for humans. The rats showed no evidence of tox-icity during the seven days they were observed. In a second study using red yeast rice extract—XueZhiKang—mice were fed an amount equivalent to a 533 times the suggested dose for humans. Again there were no signs of toxicity.

Subchronic studies use smaller doses but they are given over a greater period of time. In a subchronic test, red yeast rice was fed for ninety days to rats at dose levels of 38.5, 69.5 and 125 times the suggested human dose. Again, no toxicity was seen. This study also analyzed blood cells counts (hemoglobin, platelets, and red and white blood cells), liver enzymes, and tissue samples and found them all to be normal. A subchronic study has also been done using red yeast rice extract (XueZhiKang) and it showed similar results. Red yeast rice extract has not been shown to produce mutations and does not damage either mouse chromosomes or sperm.

In total there have been more than thirty-four clinical studies in China and the United States, and all of them have found red yeast rice and its extract to be safe and free of significant side effects.

CHINESE STUDIES

Most of the human research on red yeast rice has been done in China. Six studies included positive control groups, and of these, three compared red yeast rice extract to simvastatin, one of the statin drugs. In all three trials the extract and simvastatin were effective in improving lipid levels. In two of the studies, no significant differences were seen between the two.

In a major Chinese study that was published in 1997 in *Current Therapeutic Research*, a group of Chinese researchers compared a red yeast rice extract (Cholestin3) to another traditional treatment for high cholesterol—Jiaogulan. The Jiaogulan group was said to be a positive control group since they received another treatment. A negative control group that received a placebo was not possible in this case because Chinese guidelines would not allow it. Recipients received 14 grams of monacolins from an extract that was more concentrated than the red yeast rice powder that would be used later in the U.S. studies.

Only those volunteers with cholesterol levels greater than 229 mg/dL, LDL cholesterol greater than 129 mg/dL, and triglycerides over 200 mg/dL but less than 400 mg/dL were allowed to participate. In addition, HDL levels had to be under 40 mg/dL in men and 45 mg/dL in women. Among the 446 patients, 345 had pretreatment total cholesterol greater than 230 mg/dL. Participants who had major medical problems such as heart attack, stroke, diabetes, or a major accident or trauma were excluded. In preparation for the study, all of the patients were asked to stop any drugs they were taking for their high cholesterol. Dietary advice was then given for two to four weeks. Both the treatment and positive control groups had hyperlipidemia for the same number of years.

Finally, the study was ready to begin and the patients were divided into four groups. One group (122 men and women) received the positive control treatment—1.2 grams/day of Jiaogulan for eight weeks. The other three groups (324 men and women) received red yeast rice extract—1.2 grams/day for eight weeks. For the duration of the study patients were asked not to change their normal activities including smoking, exercise, and diet.

RESULTS OF MULTICENTER STUDY

The results of this study are summarized in Tables 5-1 and 5-2.

- Total cholesterol was reduced by an average of 17.1 percent after four weeks and 22.7 after eight weeks in the treatment group. Participants in the Jiaogulan control group experienced only a 4.8 and 7 percent decrease respectively.
- LDL cholesterol was reduced by an average of 24.6 percent after four weeks and 30.9 percent after eight weeks

in the treatment group. Reductions in the positive control group were 8.3 and 15.3 percent respectively.

- Serum triglycerides were reduced by an average of 19.8 percent after four weeks and 34.1 percent after eight weeks in the treatment group. Reductions in the positive control group were 9.2 and 12.8 percent respectively.
- HDL cholesterol was increased an average of 12.8 percent after four weeks and 19.9 percent after eight weeks. Increases in the positive control group were 4.9 and 8.4 percent respectively.

Table 5-1: Chinese Multicenter Study

	BASELINE	4 WEEKS	8 WEEKS
Total cholesterol			
Treatment	274	226	211
Positive Control	268	255	250
Triglycerides			
Treatment	273	219	178
Positive Control	273	248	238
LDL			
Treatment	186	140	127
Positive Control	180	168	165
HDL			
Treatment	36.2	40.7	43.4
Positive Control	35.5	37.1	38.5
Ratio non-HDL/HDL			
Treatment	4.86	3.61	3.19
Positive Control	5.07	4.69	4.54

The treatment group received *M. purpureus* rice preparation 1.2 grams/day containing 13.5 mg monacolins. The positive control received Jiaogulan (*Gynostemma pentaphylla*).

Table 5-2: Chinese Multicenter Study

Cholesterol over 300 mg/dL	dropped 86 mg/dL
Cholesterol under 240 mg/dL	dropped 47.1 mg/dL
LDL 130-160 mg/dL	dropped 22.4 mg/dL
LDL 200 mg/dL	dropped 34.6 mg/dL
Triglycerides over 300 mg/dL	dropped 152 mg/dL (40.1 percent)
Triglycerides under 240 mg/dL	dropped 17 mg/dL (8.8 percent)
HDL > 45 mg/dL	increased 1.81 mg/dL (4 percent)
HDL 35–45 mg/dL	increased 6.3 mg/dL (16 percent)
HDL <35 mg/dL	increased 7.9 mg/dL (25.1 percent)

The higher the cholesterol levels at the start of the study, the greater the effect of the red yeast rice extract.

But what kind of side effects were experienced? According to the authors of the study, "Severe side effects with *M.purpureus* rice treatment were rare, and the treatment was well tolerated in this study. Although mild side effects (ie, heartburn, flatulence, and dizziness) were found in a few patients, these symptoms resolved quickly."

In a second major study, 152 volunteers with cholesterol levels greater than 250 mg/dL were given a weaker form of red yeast rice that contained half the usual dose. At the end of eight weeks their total cholesterol levels were reduced by an average of 19.2 percent while the placebo group decreased only 1.5 percent. Triglycerides were reduced by an average of 36.1 percent compared to placebo of 9.15 percent. LDL cholesterol was reduced by an average of 27.1 percent and HDL was increased by 16.7 percent.

Research was presented at the American Heart Association's 39th Annual Conference on Cardiovascular Disease Epidemiology and Prevention that examined cholesterol levels in elderly men and women. Two studies were conducted in 233 elderly subjects with elevated cholesterol, which they had not been able to lower with a one-month Step I diet. Subjects who took Cholestin showed a 16.4 percent decrease in total cholesterol, a 21 percent drop in LDL-cholesterol and a 14.6 percent increase in HDL-cholesterol.

AMERICAN STUDIES

To date, two studies have been done in the United States. Both studies were financed by Pharmanex, and both lead researchers, Drs. Heber and Rippe, are members of the company's medical advisory board. Both studies also used Cholestin, a red yeast rice product that contains 4 mg HMG-CoA reductase inhibitors: 2 mg as lovastatin, 1 mg as lovastatin acid, and 1 mg as a mixture of seven other statins. This is equivalent to 7.2 mg lovastatin plus 2.4 mg of other statins for a total of 9.6 mg of monacolins.

FIRST U.S. STUDY

On April 19, 1998 at the Experimental Biology Conference, Dr. David Heber, director of the UCLA Center for Human Nutrition, presented his findings from the first U.S. clinical study on the cholesterol-lowering effects of a red yeast rice. Results were published in February, 1999, in the *Journal of*

Clinical Nutrition. Heber and company recruited eighty-three healthy volunteers—forty-six men and thirty-seven women—from newspaper advertisements and posted announcements.

Before the start of the study, both treatment and placebo groups were given instructions on how to follow the Step I diet recommended as part of the National Cholesterol Education Program and were told to maintain a 30 percent fat diet for the duration of the study. Participants were also weighed at each visit, and diet was again analyzed at the end of eight and twelve weeks. One of the goals of this study was to eliminate the possibility that the differences observed between control and treatment groups were due to changes in the participant's weight and diet.

The treatment group, who consisted of forty-two men and women, were given 1.2 grams of Cholestin a day—two 300 mg capsules twice a day. The placebo group of forty-one men and women were given look-alike capsules that contained plain rice powder.

RESULTS

Again, the results were impressive. By the end of eight weeks, blood lipid differences were already obvious and total cholesterol had decreased from an average of 254 mg/dL to 208 mg/dL in the treatment group. The placebo group, however, had no significant reduction. Participants also filled out a food frequency questionnaire. When this was analyzed it showed no significant differences between the groups. More detailed results for this study can be seen in Table 5-3. According to Dr. Heber, "In this double-blind, randomized, placebo-controlled prospective study, red yeast rice significantly reduced cholesterol concentrations, beyond effects that could be accounted for by diets alone and without significant adverse effects." HDL levels were not significantly increased, and this was believed due to the high HDL levels of participants had at the start of the study.

Table 5-3: Dr. Heber's American Study

	BASELINE	8 WEEKS	12 WEEKS
Total cholesterol			
Treatment	254	208	210
Placebo	255	254	250
Triglycerides			
Treatment	133	118	124
Placebo	143	142	146
LDL			
Treatment	173	134	135
Placebo	180	179	175
HDL			
Treatment	50	50	50
Placebo	46	46	46

SIDE EFFECTS

There were no serious side effects in any of the eighty-three participants. There were no reported adverse effects in the treatment group, while three subjects in the placebo-treated group reported minor problems. To make sure that the red yeast rice treatment was not toxic, liver and kidney function were tested at the beginning of the study and at twelve weeks. The treatment group showed no signs of toxicity. As Heber said, "There were no abnormal liver or renal function test results at any time for any subject under study."

CONCLUSIONS

The study concluded that these difference could not be due to diet alone since dietary intake and body weight were the same through out the study and no differences were found between treatment and placebo groups.

SECOND U.S. STUDY

The largest American study was directed by Dr. James Rippe of Tufts University School of Medicine in Boston. It involved primary care physicians and cardiologists from twelve medical practices across the country, including doctors from Beverly Hills, California, Chicago, Illinois, Providence, Rhode Island, Jackson Beach, Florida, and Spokane, Washington. Researchers put 233 people on Cholestin for eight weeks. The participants received 9.6 mg of monacolins a day. According to cardiologist James Rippe, M.D, lead researcher, "This is a very important study that will help millions of individuals lower their cholesterol and improve their health. Given the prevalence of cardiovascular problems in the United States, Cholestin represents an important breakthrough as a safe, effective and affordable means of achieving healthier cholesterol levels."

RESULTS

The results in this study were similar to those in Dr. Heber's. The treatment group went from an average of 274 mg/dL at the start to 226 mg/dL at the end.

- Total cholesterol fell by 16.4 percent
- LDL cholesterol fell by 21 percent
- HDL cholesterol increased by 14.6 percent

Eighteen percent reported mild to moderate side effects, mainly GI upset or headaches.

If you look closely at the data, you will notice that there is a difference between the effectiveness of the red yeast rice supplements used in China and those used in America. Although both American studies found significant reduction in total cholesterol, LDL cholesterol, and triglycerides, their effects were not as great as those found in the Chinese studies. The differences found between the Boston and Chinese study could be due to the fact that the Chinese study used a more concentrated extract while the Boston and multicenter studies used a less potent red yeast rice powder formula. Dr Rippe explained, "The Chinese study participants received approximately 13.5 milligrams of HMG-CoA reductase inhibitors each day in the Cholestin preparation they took, while the participants in the Boston study received about 9.6 mg per day."

IMPLICATIONS

But what do all these research studies mean? Yes, red yeast rice supplements lower cholesterol. But will that translate into less atherosclerosis? Fewer deaths? According to animal studies— yes. In research studies using quail and rabbits, atherosclerosis was significantly reduced in hyperlipidemic rabbits and quail after taking red yeast rice. Many large studies have been done on other statins that examine their effect on mortality.

Generally, the statins reduce the risk of heart attack by about 30 to 60 percent and the risk of death from cardiovascular disease by about 30 to 40 percent. Over a six-year period, researchers in the Scandinavian Simvastatin Survival Study group tracked more than 4,000 patients who had either survived a heart attack or been treated for angina. During that span the probability that patients taking simvastatin would die from heart disease was reduced 42 percent, while the number who had major cardiac events such as myocardial infarctions dropped 34 percent. Pooled data from four studies of pravastatin on patients suffering from heart disease showed a 62 percent reduction in the risk of heart attack.

But what about those with no history of heart disease? What benefits did the statins have to offer them? A recent study looked at 6,604 men and postmenopausal women with a mildly elevated average total cholesterol of 221 mg/dL, LDL of 150 mg/dL, and HDL 36 mg/dL. Half were given lovastatin and the other half a placebo. Overall, there were 299 cases of heart attack, serious heart pain, or fatal cardiac arrest. Women taking lovastatin had 46 percent lower risk of heart trouble than the other women. Men on the drug had a 37 percent lower risk. This has ignited a controversy. Should moderately elevated levels of cholesterol be treated with drugs? Some say yes. Others say no, stating that healthy people should not take drugs.

Perhaps the answer here is not drugs but supplements such as red yeast rice.

Cautions to Follow When Taking Red Yeast Rice

- If you take drugs to thin your blood (Warfarin or Coumadin), red yeast rice extract may increase your pro-thrombin time. Tell your physician when you start taking the supplement and be aware that you may have to adjust your dosage.
- Do not take a fiber supplement within two hours of your red yeast rice supplement.
- Do not eat grapefruit or drink grapefruit juice within two hours of your red yeast rice supplement.
- If you take any other drug, check with your physician or pharmacist before starting a red yeast rice supplement.
- It is theoretically possible for red yeast rice to lower CoQ10 levels. You may want to take a CoQ10 supplement, especially if you begin to feel tired after several months of red yeast rice supplementation.
- Take your red yeast rice supplement with meals to minimize any digestive discomfort that may occur.

6

The Red Yeast Rice Diet

Now that we understand what red yeast rice is and can do for us, we are ready to put our plan into action. There is no such thing as a miracle pill that will protect you from atherosclerosis. Red yeast rice is only going to work if it is part of an overall health plan, so you must follow this diet and a program of exercise if it is to work as designed. No supplement can overcome a diet rich in oxidized fats and cholesterol that is also devoid of antioxidants. No supplement can make up for tobacco use or a lifestyle that does not include exercise.

A Step I diet (as outlined by the American Heart Association) is not really difficult to follow. In fact, you may already be on a Step I diet and not know it. The current average American diet is estimated to include 34 percent of calories from fat, with 12 percent from saturated fat. That is just a few percentage points away from this diet. Food labels have also taken the guesswork out of food choices, and many restaurants now include nutritional information.

BEFORE YOU START YOUR DIET

Before starting this diet or any diet it is best to see your doctor. This will be a good opportunity for you to discuss your lipoprotein levels and set reasonable goals. If you have not had your cholesterol levels checked in a year, now is the time to have that done as well. You may want to bring this book with you if your doctor is not familiar with red yeast rice.

When you have your blood test results, turn to Chapter 8: *Charting Your Progress*. Record your numbers there. Take the time now to enter your weight and set weight loss goals if necessary. Use the weight chart in that chapter to calculate how many calories and how much fat your diet should be based upon. As you go through this chapter and climb the food pyramid you will be asked to compare your present diet with the recommended one. Record your present dietary habits in Chapter 8 as you are prompted at the end of each food group. This way you will have a clear idea of the specific types of dietary change you need to make.

HOW TO PURCHASE
RED YEAST RICE

Your first task is to purchase a supply of red yeast rice. I suggest that you buy a six-month supply to keep on hand. If you cannot locate red yeast rice in a store close to you, there are mail order and Internet sources listed in the back of the book. There you will also find phone numbers for those companies that take phone orders. I've found that it is cheaper to purchase many supplements this way even after you include the cost of postage.

I usually order all of my supplements on the Internet. It's a quick and easy way to comparison shop. You will find a list of my favorite mail order and Internet supplement sources in the back of the book too.

The brand of red yeast rice used in all of the studies we have discussed is called Cholestin. It is manufactured by Pharmanex Inc. of Simi Valley, California. The recommended dose of Cholestin is two 600-milligram capsules twice a day for a total of four capsules a day. A month's supply will cost you about $30 to $40. If you prefer, this company also makes a snack bar that contains one dose (1,200 mg) of Cholestin. The recommended dosage here is one bar twice a day or a combination of a bar and two capsules.

Some companies are marketing a red yeast rice product that contains a higher percentage of HMG-CoA reductase inhibitors. The number of pills you need to take is less so be sure to read the instructions on the outside of the box before you take the pill inside. The studies in the United States used 2,400 mg of red yeast rice. Do not exceed this dosage without first discussing it with your doctor.

HOW TO TAKE RED YEAST RICE

Take your red yeast rice capsules twice a day with meals. They are just as effective if taken on an empty stomach, but you increase your chances of experiencing gastrointestinal discomfort if you take them this way. Do not take your red yeast rice with grapefruit or grapefruit juice. When grapefruit juice was taken with lovastatin, a HMG-CoA reductase inhibitor, it caused a fifteen-fold increase in serum concentrations of lovastatin and its active breakdown product, lovastatin acid. This is an overdose. Enjoy your grapefruit either two hours before or after you take your supplement.

THE DIET PLAN

This diet is a whole foods version of the American Heart Association's Step I diet. It emphasizes whole foods over refined products and unprocessed or minimally processed foods over prepared, processed foods.

- **30 percent** of the day's total calories should come from fat.
- **50 to 55 percent** of the day's total calories should come from carbohydrate.
- **15 percent** of the day's total calories should come from protein.
- Consume just enough calories to achieve and maintain a healthy weight.

You should eat 25 to 30 grams of fiber a day from food. It is allright to get a few grams from supplements, but most should come from whole grains, fruits, and vegetables. Most Americans eat only 15 grams of fiber a day, half of the recommended amount.

Food-wise, the above translates into these recommendations:

Table 6-1

FOOD GROUP	SUGGESTED SERVINGS
Vegetables	4-6 servings
Fruits	3-5 servings
Breads, cereals, rice, potatoes, and pasta	6-11 servings
Milk, yogurt, and cheese	2-3 servings
Meats, poultry, fish, dry beans and peas, eggs, and nuts (at least 2 servings of cold water fish a week)	2-3 servings

Each day you should eat this many servings. How you distribute them throughout the day is up to you. Remember, too many carbohydrates will increase your blood sugar levels, which can adversely affect your triglycerides. To reduce this effect of carbohydrates, eat some protein or fat with each serving.

Eat a variety of foods daily, choosing different foods from each group. The larger number of servings are for those with high-calorie diets. If you need to gain weight, increase the amount of servings you eat. If you need to lose weight, decrease your serving size.

Sources of Soluble Fiber

Soluble fiber has been shown to reduce cholesterol levels. Enjoy at least two servings of these foods each day.

- Oat bran
- Rice bran
- Oatmeal—avoid the quick cooking types; they can elevate your blood sugar
- Cold oat cereals—avoid those with added sugar

- Barley
- Ground flaxseed
- Ground psyllium seed (found in some natural laxatives)

CLIMBING THE PYRAMID

I have found that most people do not really understand what percentages mean. I prefer to use the food pyramid with its food groups. The groups are easier to understand and put into action. Take a good look at the food pyramid in Figure 6-1. The base of the pyramid is the bread, cereal, rice, potato, and pasta group. When eaten whole, these foods provide you with energy in the form of carbohydrates, the B complex vitamins, and minerals. On the next step are the fruit and vegetable group. When I was a child, both fruits and vegetables shared a single group. As our understanding of the roles these foods play in good health has increased, so has the recommended number of servings. Fruits and vegetables now occupy a much more prominent position.

On the third rung are the dairy and protein groups. I have added another group to this level, the soy group. Soy foods are an important part of a healthy diet. At the very top is the fats, oils, and sweets group. In addition to the obvious foods in this group—fat, oil, and sugar—I have added junk food and fast food. As we have seen, fast food poses one of the biggest threats to your cardiovascular health.

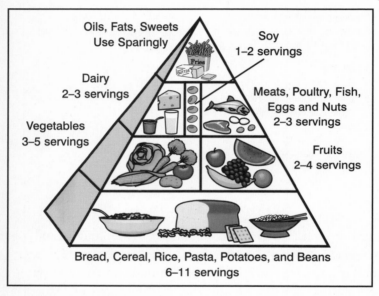

Figure 6-1. Food Pyramid

According to University of Michigan researchers, a low fat diet is not always best.

They examined the overall diet of men and women in the United States based on diet diversity (consuming foods from the five major food groups), variety (total number of foods consumed per day), and moderation (following USDA food guidelines). The team examined the eating habits of 1,637 men and 1,576 women over two days and then compared those results to a Paris study that examined the eating habits of 5,000 French adults.

French men and women ate more foods higher in fat, saturated fat, and cholesterol than the Americans, meeting few of the USDA recommendations for healthy eating. The study concluded that 99 percent of the French

THE BREAD, CEREAL, RICE, PASTA, POTATO, AND BEAN GROUP

The very base of the food pyramid is the bread, cereal, rice, potato, and bean group. Base your diet on these foods with six to eleven servings each day.

One serving equals:

- 1 slice of bread
- 1/2 bun, bagel, or English muffin
- 1 ounce of dry ready-to-eat cereal
- 1/2 cup of cooked cereal, rice, pasta, or potatoes
- 1 medium whole potato
- 1/2 cup of cooked dry beans, peas, or lentils

This group supplies your body with complex carbohydrates, trace minerals, protein, and fiber. You should base your diet on these foods. However, many folks misinterpret this recommendation to mean a diet based on whole wheat—for example pasta, bread, or cereals. Complex carbohydrates are more than just wheat. Expand your culinary horizons and eat a variety of carbs. Oats are a good choice because they lower cholesterol levels. Brown rice is also a good choice.

women derived more than 10 percent of their calories from saturated fat. Despite this, the French have fewer cases of heart disease and are less obese than Americans.

The higher intake of fat in the French diet was balanced by greater dietary diversity and variety. Researchers found that those people who had more diversity in their diets consumed more calories, fat, saturated fat, cholesterol, and fiber. Typically, men had more diverse diets than women, and elderly women consumed the least fat and had much less diverse diets. Only one in ten men and one in sixteen women consumed at least one serving of each of the five good groups—meat, dairy, grains, vegetables, and fruits—over two days.

LEGUMES

Most food pyramids put legumes higher up on the pyramid with the other protein foods. While legumes are rich protein sources, they are also excellent sources of fiber and carbohydrates. They belong on the bottom of the pyramid. Eat them at least five times a week, including beans such as soy beans, adzuki beans, lima beans, black beans, black-eyed peas, brown beans, pinto beans, red beans, fava beans, kidney beans, navy beans, white beans, and chick peas, lentils, split peas, and green peas. Add beans to soups and stews. A large bowl of split pea soup makes a satisfying lunch that won't let you slump in the afternoon.

A large recent study of men found that for every extra ten grams of fiber eaten, a man's risk of dying from heart disease dropped by 17 percent. In a six-year study of 21,930 Finnish men aged fifty to sixty-nine, researchers found that for each additional ten grams of fiber consumed daily (about three slices of rye bread), a man's risk of dying from MI dropped 17 percent.

The average U.S. male eats only seventeen grams of fiber each day, about two-thirds that of the average Finn.

WHOLE GRAIN BENEFITS

Each grain has its own unique blend of fibers, vitamins, and minerals that can help to prevent atherosclerosis.

- Wheat, oats, and barley contain arginine, an amino acid that helps the arteries to relax, reducing the risk of heart disease, hypertension, and stroke.
- Brown rice contains beta sitosterol, a phytosterol also found in red yeast rice. It will help to decrease cholesterol absorption in the intestine.
- Oats and quinoa contain saponins, compounds that lower cholesterol and have an antibiotic effect.

- Brown rice, oats, and barley contain tocotrienol, a form of vitamin E that may be able to reduce cholesterol production.
- Barley, oats, and particularly oat bran contain beta glucan, a type of soluble fiber that decreases cholesterol.
- Amaranth contains squalene, another lipid that inhibits HMG-CoA reductase like red yeast rice.
- Wheat germ, amaranth, triticale, rye, millet, and wild rice contain folate, a B vitamin that reduces serum homocysteine levels.
- Amaranth, rye, oats, whole wheat, and especially wheat germ contain vitamin E, a fat-soluble antioxidant that may reduce plaque levels and hypertension and prevent strokes.
- Wheat germ, buckwheat, millet, quinoa, brown rice, rye, triticale, and amaranth all contain magnesium, a mineral that reduces vasoconstriction and reduces blood pressure and platelet stickiness.

In a study funded by Quaker Oats, Tufts University researchers compared a study group given an oat-rich diet to a control group given a wheat-rich diet. At the end of the study, participants on the oat diet had lower blood pressure and reduced blood levels of cholesterol. The oat diet lowered total blood cholesterol by 34 milligrams per deciliter (mg/dL) while the control diet lowered cholesterol levels by only 13 mg/dL. The individuals' blood levels of low-density lipoprotein cholesterol (LDL) followed the same pattern: The oat group's LDL was 23 mg/dL lower and the wheat group's LDL was 8 mg/dL lower.

Participants in the oat group also reduced their systolic (top number) blood pressure by 7 millimeters of mercury (mm Hg) at the end of the six-week study compared to 2 mm Hg for the wheat group.

The two diets differed mainly in the amount of soluble fiber. Oats contain more of this fiber than the same quantity of wheat. Other foods high in soluble fiber are barley, lentils, pinto beans, black beans, and citrus fruits.

FOODS TO EMPHASIZE

Whole grains such as amaranth, barley, buckwheat, corn, Kamut, millet, oats, quinoa, brown rice, rye, spelt, triticale, wheat, and wild rice; whole grain products such as pasta, breads, crackers, and flours; cereals such as hot and cold cereal; brans such as oat, rice, and wheat bran; and germs such as wheat and rice polish.

Researchers at the University of Minnesota Heart Disease Prevention Clinic showed that eating one and a half ounces of Cheerios twice a day lowered cholesterol levels of study participants by an average of 3.8 percent, but Cheerios lowered cholesterol for some participants by as much as 18 percent.

For a twelve-week period, 135 men and women were given either an unidentified whole-grain oat cereal (Cheerios) to eat daily or an unidentified corn flake cereal. On average, those who ate Cheerios achieved a significant reduction in blood cholesterol while those who ate the corn flakes did not.

"After I began eating Cheerios for the study, my cholesterol dropped by 40 points," said one study participant.

FOODS TO AVOID

- Limit your intake of all refined grains including white flour and white rice. Once or twice a week for a treat is fine, but be careful they do not become a habit.
- The same advice goes for cakes, cookies, pies, and muffins because these foods also contain large amounts of fat. Put a piece of pie on a paper towel and see how much fat leaks into the paper!
- Choose long cooking oatmeal (over five minutes) rather than the quick cooking, which will raise your glucose levels.
- Be aware of the so-called healthy bakery products such as bran muffins and cookies. Get your fiber some other less fatty way.

Whole Grain Oat Fact Sheet

- Oat consumption by humans dates back to 400 B.C. when oats were described as a "healing agent."
- Oats came to America in 1602 and were used for relief of stomach discomforts and other ailments.
- Whole grain oats contain more soluble fiber than other whole grains such as wheat, corn, or rye.
- Whole grain oats contain more protein and lipids than other grains.
- Oats contain naturally occurring phytochemicals that have been associated with protection from a variety of chronic diseases. Whole grains contain naturally occurring phytoestrogens, which have been linked to decreased risk of hormone-related diseases such as breast cancer.
- Scientists first discovered oats lowered cholesterol in 1963.
- Oats are a good source of selenium, iron, calcium, manganese, magnesium, zinc, and copper.
- Oats are concentrated sources of antioxidants, which are thought to decrease the risk of cancer and aging, according to the American Oat Association.

FOODS TO ELIMINATE

Any foods fried in hot oil such as donuts and fried pies. They can be sources of oxidized fats.

Your servings of the bread, cereal, rice, potato, and bean group:

I now eat this many servings: _____
Now turn to Chapter 8 and record your intake and goals.

FRUIT GROUP

The fruit group shares a level with the vegetable group on the next rung up from breads and cereals. Have at least two to four servings of fruit each day. Half your servings may be juiced.

One serving equals:

- 1 medium piece of fruit
- 1/2 cup of small diced fruit
- 3/4 cup of juice

BENEFITS OF FRUIT

Almost all fruits are excellent sources of potassium. This mineral increases the removal of sodium from the body and reduces blood pressure in those with hypertension. One of the reasons hypertension is so common today is due to the lack of fruits and vegetables in the typical American diet.

- Pears, oranges, and cantaloupe are good sources of the B vitamin folate. Low folate levels increase the amount of a chemical called homocysteine circulating in the blood. Homocysteine is toxic to the endothelium and is linked with an increased chance of developing heart disease.
- Berries such as strawberries, blueberries, blackberries, cranberries, and raspberries contain salicylates, a natural form of aspirin that may be able to reduce inflammation and reduce blood coagulation. Their bright colors come from the flavonoid pigments in their cells. These pigments act as antioxidants. A study of 5,133 Finns found that those whose diets were highest in flavonoids were less likely to die from coronary artery disease than those whose diets contained less flavonoids. Blueberries also contain saponins, which may reduce cholesterol levels, and strawberries are rich in vitamin C, needed to recycle vitamin E.
- Strawberries are also a good choice. Researchers gave eight elderly women a special beverage made with strawberry juices. They found that it boosted the women's ability to fight off oxidation as much as a 1,250 mg dose of vitamin C!
- Fresh pineapple contains the protein-digesting enzyme bromelain, which may reduce platelet aggregation. Cantaloupe also appears to contain substances that decrease the viscosity of the blood.

- Watermelon, dried apricots, pink grapefruit, guava, and papaya are good sources of lycopene, a major carotenoid pigment. Although the role of lycopene in risk reduction of cardiovascular disease remains unclear, lower concentrations of lycopene have been found in people with elevated cholesterol.

A daily glass of purple grape juice may help prevent cardiovascular disease, according to Wisconsin researchers. In two small studies of healthy subjects and rhesus monkeys they found that drinking three glasses of purple grape juice a day was about as protective as a daily aspirin for patients with heart disease. The grape juice did this by reducing platelet aggregation by about 40 percent.

No such effects were found with orange and grapefruit juice. Purple grape juice contains a certain type of flavonoid that is absent in orange and grapefruit juice.

FOODS TO EMPHASIZE IN THE FRUIT GROUP

Fruits rich in soluble fiber such as apples, pears, strawberries, and citrus fruits (oranges, lemons, grapefruit, tangerines); flavonoid-rich fruits such as blueberries, blackberries, cherries, and raspberries; carotene-rich fruits such as all orange and red colored fruits including apricots, cantaloupe, mangoes, papayas, peaches, and watermelon; all other fresh and frozen fruits including bananas, plums, kiwi, and honeydew melon; dried fruit such as figs, dates, raisins, and prunes; fruit canned in juice or water; applesauce and other stewed fruit without added sugar; fruit juice without added sugar; and orange juice fortified with calcium.

Your servings of the fruit group:

I now eat this many servings: _____
Now turn to Chapter 8 and record your intake and goals.

VEGETABLE GROUP

Sharing the same level as the fruit group is the vegetable group. Eat at least three to five servings of these foods each day. Up to two servings may be juiced.

One serving equals:

- 1 cup of raw leafy greens
- 1/2 cup cooked greens
- 1/2 cup chopped vegetable
- 1 medium vegetable

The following foods when fresh or frozen are rich in glutathione. Canned, bottled, or cooked foods contain little glutathione since this important nutrient is destroyed by heat. Glutathione is an important antioxidant that protects your endothelium.

- Asparagus, tops and bottom
- Avocados
- Brussels sprouts
- Broccoli, stem and flower
- Cabbage
- Cauliflower
- Grapefruit
- Okra
- Oranges
- Peaches
- Strawberries
- Squash
- Tomatoes
- Watermelon
- White potatoes

In general, emphasize the vegetables rich in the protective antioxidants. If fresh or frozen vegetables are not available, you can eat those canned without added salt, fat, or sugar. Canned or bottled tomato sauce is fine and is a good source of the antioxidant lycopene. If you have your own juicer you can juice up to two servings of vegetables.

Vegetables are wonderful sources of carbohydrates, vitamins, minerals, and fiber. They also contain so many phytonutrients—plant chemicals that act as nutrients—I couldn't list them all. Here is a sampling.

- Brussels sprouts, cabbage, leek, parsley, celery, and especially onion are sources of polyphenols—substances that act as antioxidants and free radical scavengers. Epidemiologic studies have shown a correlation between an increased consumption of phenolic antioxidants and a reduced risk of cardiovascular disease.
- Tomatoes in any form—fresh, cooked, canned, juiced, and as catsup—are a good source of lycopene, a major carotenoid pigment. Although the role of lycopene in risk reduction of cardiovascular disease remains unclear, lower concentrations of lycopene have been found in people with elevated cholesterol.
- Shitake, Maitake, and Reishi mushrooms are able to lower lipids levels and high blood pressure.
- Cruciferous vegetables including broccoli, Brussels sprouts, cabbage, bok choy, kale, collard and mustard greens, and cauliflower contain the antioxidants vitamin C and beta carotene and are good sources of soluble and insoluble fiber.
- Sweet peppers and turnip greens are also good sources of the antioxidant vitamin C, which is necessary to recycle vitamin E.
- Garlic, onions, leeks, and shallots contains organosulfur compounds, which may help prevent thrombi from forming.

FOODS TO EMPHASIZE IN THE VEGETABLE GROUP

All fresh and frozen vegetables including yellow, red, and orange vegetables (carotene sources) such as yams, sweet potatoes, carrots, pumpkin, winter squash, rutabaga, tomatoes, red bell peppers, and corn; green leafy vegetables such as turnip greens, mustard greens, collards, green and red loose-leaf lettuce, romaine, butter lettuce, escarole, chicory, dandelion greens, and sorrel; cruciferous vegetables such as Brussels sprouts, cauliflower, kale, cabbage, and bok choy; sprouts such as bean sprouts and alfalfa sprouts; and all other vegetable such as green pea, asparagus, and green bell peppers.

Avoid frozen vegetable combinations that contain sauces made with fats containing trans fatty acids or cheese sauces made with dried cheese and milk that contain oxidized fats and cholesterol. Read labels!

Your servings of the vegetable group:

I now eat this many servings: _____
Now turn to Chapter 8 and record your intake and goals.

DAIRY GROUP

On the third level of the food pyramid we have the dairy foods. This group contains all milk products including milk, sour cream, cream, yogurt, cheese, cottage cheese, and butter. Eat two to three servings of this group or another calcium-rich food each day

One serving equals:

- 1 cup of milk or yogurt
- 1½ ounces of cheese

Milk products can be a protein source, but they are given their own group because of their calcium content. Many people do not drink milk because they are allergic to its proteins, intolerant of its sugar (lactose intolerance), or just don't like the taste. If you do not drink milk be careful to get enough calcium. For alternate calcium sources see the list of calcium-rich foods in Chapter 7. The best milk "replacement" is fortified fresh soy milk, which also contains a variety of other heart protective substances.

Whole milk products contain a large amount of saturated fat. This makes it a good choice for very young children with high energy needs and developing nervous systems that need cholesterol. But adults need to limit their consumption. The saturated fat in milk will also increase your LDL levels without providing the antioxidants needed to protect them. Unprotected high LDL levels translate into atherosclerosis and all the diseases that implies. If you consume a lot of milk fat you should take an antioxidant supplement (see Chapter 7 for instructions on how to pick one).

DAIRY PRODUCTS TO ELIMINATE

The cholesterol in milk is also prone to oxidation. Eliminate all milk products that have been exposed to high temperatures or dried, including powdered or dried eggs, egg yolks, butter, whole milk, or cheese. These dried milk products are often used in dry sauce mixes and as coatings or flavorings in a wide variety of processed foods. Dried or instant nonfat milk and milk products are OK since they do not contain fat or cholesterol.

This processing causes the cholesterol to oxidize. The oxidized cholesterol you eat is built into your LDL particles where it initiates or accelerates atherosclerosis. For more information on oxidation read Chapters 2 and 3. Since it is impossible to eliminate oxidized fats and cholesterol completely, make sure you eat plenty of fruit and vegetables to protect your cells.

DAIRY PRODUCTS TO AVOID

Also avoid cream, whipping cream, sour cream, coffee cream, whole milk, and other whole milk products. These can be a source of calories and saturated fat, which can increase your cholesterol levels. Researchers think that high levels of cholesterol may increase the density of red blood cell membranes, making it more difficult for oxygen to enter the cell. This means red blood cells may not be able to take on enough oxygen in the blood or deliver adequate amounts to the heart and other tissues.

THE RED YEAST RICE CHOLESTEROL SOLUTION

Ice cream, cheesecake, custard, and other full-fat desserts also contain large amounts of sugar. A dab or tablespoon of cream now and then won't hurt you, but if you make these foods a habit they will expand your waistline and possibly put you at risk for heart disease.

DAIRY PRODUCTS TO LIMIT

Desserts made with dairy foods are more sweets than nutrient sources. Limit your intake of low-fat or fat-free ice cream, artificial and low-fat whipping creams and the desserts that contain them, and nonfat yogurt or other dairy products sweetened with Nutrasweet.

FOODS TO EMPHASIZE IN THE DAIRY GROUP

Yogurt made with live cultures (check the label, it will tell you) including low-fat, nonfat, plain, and flavored; milk including low-fat, nonfat, and skim, buttermilk, Acidophilus; low-fat cheeses; cottage cheese including flavored and plain nonfat or low-fat; low-fat and nonfat sour cream; and nonfat powdered or instant milk and milk products (check the label to be sure no fats have been added to the product).

Your servings of the dairy group:

I now eat this many servings: _____
Now turn to Chapter 8 and record your intake and goals.

THE PROTEIN GROUP—MEATS, POULTRY, FISH, EGGS, NUTS AND SEEDS

Also on the third level are the protein foods. This large group includes meats, poultry, fish, eggs, and nuts and seeds. Eat two to three servings a day.

108

One serving equals:

- 6 ounces of meat or fish (about the size of a deck of cards)
- 1 cup of milk or yogurt
- 1½ ounces of cheese
- 3 ounces of tofu
- 3 ounces of nut butter such as peanut butter
- 1 egg

This group supplies protein, a nutrient necessary for the repair and maintenance of tissues. Protein is found in almost all foods. The richest source is muscle meat. Although we tend to think of animal protein as superior to plant protein, this is not true. Animal protein comes packaged with lots of fat, few vitamins and minerals, and no fiber while plant protein is accompanied by lots of vitamins, minerals, and fiber. If you are a vegetarian, don't worry about eating complementary amino acids at each meal. As long as you are getting enough calories you are probably eating enough protein.

FISH

Fish are an excellent source of low-fat protein. Some epidemiologic data suggest that consumption of fish of any type, seemingly independent of omega-3 fatty acids, is associated with reduced CHD risk. Eat at least two to three servings a week.

Fish are not only sources of protein, they also bring the healthful omega-3 fatty acids. Choose cold water fish as often as you can, including herring, sardine, anchovy, mackerel, salmon, and trout. Always eat the skin; it contains valuable oils. Avoid deep fried fish fillets that may contain oxidized fats.

Individuals who eat fish regularly are at lower risk of fatal myocardial infarction than those who do not eat fish at all.

Researchers followed a group of 1,822 Chicago men. Of those, 293 died of heart attacks, 430 from any type of coronary artery disease, 573 from cardiovascular disease, and 1,042 from any cause. Compared with those who ate no fish, those who reported eating two servings of fish a week were almost half as likely to die from a heart attack.

Since the level of omega-3 fatty acids in a weekly diet that includes thirty-five grams a day of fish may not be high enough to be effective, there may be other unidentified substances in fish that provide health benefits.

MEAT

When I was a child, each meal was built around meat. It was offered three times a day: breakfast meat, lunch meat, and dinner meat. Meat in itself is not bad, it's just that we tend to go overboard and eat it all the time. Our serving sizes are also too large. A single serving of meat (which is six ounces) is only the size of a deck of cards. If you are eating meat at a meal most people would eat twice that amount—two servings. A good size steak is twelve ounces—four servings. Combine this with the other meat we eat during the day and all the other sources of protein we eat (milk, eggs, etc.) and you can see why some researchers claim we eat too much protein. Meat (even red meat) does not need to be eliminated. It just needs to be put into its proper place and eaten in moderation. You can do this by changing the types of meat you eat, eating meat less often, and eating less when it is served.

- Limit yourself to one six-ounce serving of low-fat meat a day.
- Have at least one meatless meal a week.
- Poultry should always be eaten with the skin removed to reduce calories.

- Choose the leaner (and more flavorful and cheaper) beef cuts and cook them quickly in a pressure cooker. Remove any obvious fat from the meat.
- Recommended meats include: poultry such as chicken, duck, pheasant, game hen, emu, and ostrich; lean beef such as round, sirloin, chuck, loin; leaner "choice" or "select" grades of beef; lean or extra lean ground beef (no more than 15% fat); lean ham and pork such as tenderloin and loin chop; lean lamb such as leg, arm, and loin; and wild game such as rabbit and venison.
- Avoid processed meats such as hot dogs, sausage, meat sticks and jerky, and those found in the deli; prime grades of beef; and deep fried meats.

NUTS AND SEEDS

Nuts and seeds are good sources of protein, but since they are also rich in calories you should limit their consumption unless you are trying to gain weight. Nuts are good sources of fiber and heart healthy fats. Recommended nuts include: all fresh and dry roasted nuts such as almonds, Brazil nuts, cashews, filberts, pecans, pine nuts, pistachios, and walnuts; fresh unseasoned seeds such as pumpkin seeds, sesame seeds, sunflower seeds, and flaxseed; nut and seed butters such as tahini or sesame seed butter, walnut butter, almond butter, hazelnut butter, cashew butter, and sunflower butter; and nut milks such as almond and cashew milk. Psyllium seed husk powder is an especially rich source of soluble fiber; however, it must always be mixed with a liquid. It is tasteless so it mixes easily with juice.

Nuts and seeds are sources of:

- Arginine, a precursor to nitric oxide, a compound that relaxes the artery walls.

- Vitamin E, an antioxidant that prevents the formation of oxidized LDL
- Folic acid to help lower homocysteine levels
- Copper and magnesium, which protect from heart disease, hypertension, and stroke
- Alpha linolenic acid, high levels of which are associated with lower risk of stroke
- Monounsaturated fats, which have a positive effect on serum lipids
- Fiber, which is associated with a lower risk of cardiovascular disease

In the Harvard investigation linking nut consumption to a reduced risk of heart disease, alpha-linolenic acid, a component of nuts, may protect the heart by preventing a rhythm disturbance called ventricular fibrillation that causes sudden death. When the heart lapses into ventricular fibrillation, it cannot pump blood unless shocked into a normal rhythm with an electrical device called a defibrillator.

Other sources of alpha-linolenic acid are unhydrogenated canola and soybean oils used in most full-fat commercial salad dressings, flaxseed and flaxseed oil, and a leafy vegetable called smooth purslane eaten mainly in Greece.

Those questioned who ate the highest amount of nuts had the lowest risk for any heart-related death—even after adjusting for age, exercise habits, high blood pressure, cholesterol levels, diabetes, alcohol use, other dietary habits, and whether individuals were being treated for heart disease.

Avoid:

- nut and seed butters with hydrogenated oils that contain trans fatty acids
- nuts cooked in hot oils

Your servings of the meats, poultry, fish, eggs, and nuts and seeds group:

I now eat this many servings: _____

Now turn to Chapter 8 and record your intake and goals.

SOY FOODS

Soy foods are not part of the official pyramid, but because they can have such profound affects on your health I have included them here. Eat at least one serving of soy foods each day. Soy foods include soy milk, soybeans, tofu, tempeh, miso, soy nuts, soy flour, soy protein, soy grits, soy cheese, and edamame.

Soy foods can substitute for servings in the grain and legume group or meat group, fortified soy milk can substitute for servings in the milk group, and green soybeans (edamame) can substitute for servings in the vegetables. What a versatile food!

Soy foods are all made from the soybean. This legume is rich in protein—fourteen grams of high-quality protein in a one-half cup serving of cooked mature soybeans. But soy products are much more than just a good source of nutrients; they contain a number of substances that are good for your heart. It has been estimated that just one cup of soybeans or twenty-five grams of soy protein can lower cholesterol levels by 10 to 15 percent in persons with elevated cholesterol.

Table 6-2: Protein Content of Some Soy Foods

SOY FOOD	GRAMS OF PROTEIN
Soybeans, 1/2 cup cooked	14
Soy milk, 1 cup	7
Roasted soy nuts, 1/2 cup	34
Soy flour, 1/4 cup	8
Tempeh, 1/2 cup	16
Textured soy protein, 1/2 cup	11
Tofu, 1/2 cup	10

Phytosterols, such as beta sitosterol, are found in high concentration in soy products. Plant sterols resemble cholesterol in their chemical makeup and compete with dietary cholesterol for absorption in the small intestine. Saponins, also found in soy, act as antioxidants and bind cholesterol. Red yeast rice contains both saponins and a number of phytosterols.

Soy contains isoflavones, a substance unique to soybeans. In addition to being antioxidants, isoflavones lower total serum cholesterol and LDL cholesterol, and increase the HDL to LDL ratio. Injured endothelial cells attract white blood cells, which then stick to the vessel walls and divide. These cells then penetrate the wall and contribute to plaque growth. Genistein, an isoflavone, prevents white blood cells from sticking to the cell wall and from multiplying. It has also been found to inhibit the platelet activation that contributes to thrombi (blood clots).

Soy milk makes an excellent milk replacement. Chose a soy milk that is fortified with vitamin D, calcium, and riboflavin. Soy milk naturally contains no cholesterol and very little saturated fat. The PUFAs it does contain are protected from oxidation by several antioxidants.

According to research performed at Wake Forest University Baptist Medical Center, the isoflavones found in soy can lower serum cholesterol levels.

Researchers studied the effects of isoflavones, the compound in soybeans associated with their ability to lower cholesterol levels. The study population of 156 patients had an average total cholesterol of 241 and an average LDL cholesterol of 164, both of which are considered moderately elevated.

Patients were given soy drinks containing 25 mg of soy protein from identical containers with either 25, 42, or 58 milligrams of isoflavone or a soy drink without isoflavones. Another group of patients got a beverage containing only casein, the principal protein of cow's milk.

Soy drinks containing isoflavones reduced both total cholesterol and LDL. In patients who started with a high LDL cholesterol, the effect was even more dramatic: a 10 percent reduction in just nine weeks. The study produced stepwise results: the higher the concentration of isoflavones, the greater the reduction in both total and LDL cholesterol.

Those who drank the soy drink that lacked isoflavones or the casein drink had no such effect.

Soy milk is available in a wide variety of forms. Fresh soy milk, which you can find in the dairy case, is superior in taste to soy milk sold in aseptic packages (the kind that do not need refrigeration). The high heat treatment given to milk packaged this way changes the flavor, giving it a slight "beany" taste. If you have never tasted soy milk before, you might want to start with the fresh flavored kinds and serve them well chilled.

Enjoy all soy foods: soy milk including regular, low-fat, nonfat, fortified, vanilla, chocolate, and carob; tofu including flavored, soft, firm; tempeh; soy nuts; soy flour, soy grits; soy cheese; edamame; and miso.

Your servings of the soybean group:

I now eat this many servings: _____
Now turn to Chapter 8 and record your intake and goals.

FATS AND OILS

At the very top of the pyramid we find the most concentrated sources of energy—fats and oils. Limit your consumption to five to eight servings a day including the fats used in cooking and seasoning.

One serving equals:

- 1 teaspoon butter, oil, margarine
- 2 teaspoons mayonnaise or nut butters
- 1 tablespoon salad dressing
- 1 tablespoon cream cheese
- 2 teaspoons low-fat margarine or spread
- 3 teaspoons seeds or nuts
- 1/8 medium avocado
- 10 small or 5 large olives

RECOMMENDED FATS AND OILS

Choose oils that contain a high percentage of monounsaturated fats such as olive, almond, avocado, macadamia, and hazelnut oils that are cold pressed oils and minimally processed. Canola oil is a good choice for cooking. If you must use a margarine, buy a soft tub, liquid margarine, or spread. These have a lower percentage of hydrogenated oils and less trans fatty acids. Butter is fine for occasional use. However, use only one pat per roll or potato. It is not wise to drench your food in any kind of fat. Mayonnaise is almost all fat, so use it sparingly and buy a brand that contains only canola oil.

These oils can usually be found in health food stores and some supermarkets. A good oil will usually identify itself by its packaging. They are usually sold in small quantities so you do not have to store them for long. Good oils should be stored in the refrigerator.

- Extra virgin olive oil
- Cold pressed canola oil
- Cold pressed nut oils such as walnut or macadamia nut oil

Oils rich in essential fatty acids such as flaxseed oil are fragile and should be packaged in dark bottles, which reduces their exposure to light.

Most of the fats that you eat will be hidden inside of prepared or processed foods. High-fat foods include bakery goods, cakes, cookies, pies, muffins, and donuts and those with cheese. Always check the label of prepared foods to identify those that are high in fat. Never make high-fat foods a habit. Save them for occasional treats.

Remember: 1 tablespoon equals 3 teaspoons. The common teaspoon you have at home holds more than the standard teaspoon used to measure foods. Find out how much your teaspoons and tablespoons at home hold so you have a quick way to measure always at hand.

Butter is a dairy product, but I have included it here as a fat because it contains butterfat. Butter is a rich source of cholesterol. I am very pro-butter. It is a natural product that does not contain dangerous trans or oxidized fats like many so called "healthy" margarines and spreads. It is a source of vitamin A and of a fat called conjugated linoleic acid (CLA), which may decrease your risk of atherosclerosis as well as increase muscle weight. Our low-fat diets contain 80 percent less CLA than they did twenty years ago.

Look for oils that are unrefined and cold pressed. If you need a refined oil to use in cooking, find a brand that is minimally processed with no solvents used and no artificial preservatives added.

Respect your oils and treat them gently. They contain fragile polyunsaturated fatty acids that are easily broken down by oxygen and other free radicals such as the ultraviolet light in daylight. Store your oils in the refrigerator or in a cool place away from light. Buy them in small quantities and use before they become rancid. The oils sold in large plastic containers are the nutritional equivalent of white rice. They lack the fragrant taste of unrefined oils. A good oil does not need to be used in large quantities.

OILS AND FATS TO USE IN MODERATION

- Fresh butter
- Better Butter (recipe can be found in Chapter 7)
- Mayonnaise and salad dressings made with the above oils
- Margarines that contain liquid vegetable oil as the first ingredient (low in trans fats)

- Lowfat dressings
- Benecol

FATS AND OIL TO LIMIT

- Hydrogenated fats such as vegetable shortening and stick margarines.
- Highly refined oils.

FATS AND OILS TO AVOID

- Oils heated to high temperatures for deep frying
- Ghee (butter that has been heated to high temperatures)
- Dried butter

The types of fatty acids that are found in various fats can be seen in Table 6-3. Saturated fats are stable and will not become oxidated when heated to high temperatures. However, they can cause your normal LDL levels to rise. Polyunsaturated fatty acids are needed since they contain the essential fatty acids. However, these fats are very fragile and easily oxidize. Monounsaturated fatty acids are more stable to heat.

- Canola oil is a good choice because it is low in PUFAs while being rich in the EFAs. It also contains a high percentage of the more stable monounsaturates.
- Olive oil is a good choice because it is so stable (a high percentage of monounsaturates and saturates—87 percent). Extra virgin olive also contain important antioxidants.

Your servings of the oil and fat group:

I now eat this many servings: _____
Now turn to Chapter 8 and record your intake and goals.

Table 6-3: Oils and Fats

	PUFAs*	MUFA*	Total	SFAs*
Unsaturated*				
Safflower Oil	75%	12%	86%	9%
Sunflower Oil	66%	20%	86%	10%
Corn Oil	59%	24%	83%	13%
Soybean Oil	58%	23%	81%	14%
Cottonseed Oil	52%	18%	70%	26%
Canola Oil**	33%	55%	88%	7%
Olive Oil	8%	74%	82%	13%
Peanut Oil	32%	46%	78%	17%
Soft Tub Margarine***	31%	47%	78%	17%
Palm Oil	9%	37	46%	49%
Coconut Oil	2%	6%	8%	86%
Palm Kernel Oil	2%	11%	13%	81%
Animal Fats				
Tuna Fat****	37%	26%	63%	27%
Chicken Fat	21%	45%	66%	30%
Lard	11%	45%	56%	40%
Mutton Fat	8%	41%	49%	47%
Beef Fat	4%	42%	46%	50%
Butter Fat	4%	29%	33%	62%

* Values are given as a percent of total fat.
** Canola oil is a good choice because it is low in PUFAs while being right in EFAs. It also contains a high percentage of the more stable monounsaturates.
*** Made with hydrogenated soybean oil plus hydrogenated cottonseed oil.
**** Fat from white tuna, canned in water, solids drained.

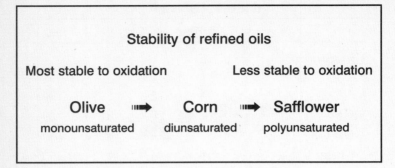

Figure 6-2 Oils vary in stability.

Olive oil contains triglycerides that contain a high percentage of MUFAs, corn oil contains a high percentage of triglycerides that contain diunsaturates, and safflower oil contains triglycerides that contain a high percentage of PUFAs. In their unrefined or virgin state these oils contain antioxidants, mainly vitamin E. In fact, the amount of vitamin E in a given oil is proportional to its PUFA content. Unfortunately, we usually consume refined oils that have been stripped of their antioxidants. The result is fatty acids in our diet and bodies that are prone to oxidation.

7

Diet Tips

Whenever a person tries to change his or her pattern of eating, he or she is bound to have lots of questions. Hopefully the following questions and answers will help you to follow your new eating plan. They will help you plan your meals and introduce variety into them, choose a food supplement, and understand antioxidants.

FREQUENTLY ASKED QUESTIONS ABOUT RED YEAST RICE

What is red yeast rice?

The scientific name for red yeast rice is *Monascus purpureus* rice, and it is made from the strain of *M. purpureus* Went yeast. In Chinese it is called Hung-chu or Hong Qu. Red yeast rice has been used for centuries in China to make rice wine, as a food preservative for maintaining the color and taste of fish and meat, and for medicinal properties. In the United States it is sold under a number of brand names including Cholestin, the brand used in all American research.

How long will it take for my cholesterol levels to drop?

In studies, a significant reduction was seen after four weeks with maximum effect occurring after two months.

How does red yeast rice work?

The key ingredients in red yeast rice are substances called HMG-CoA reductase inhibitors. Red yeast rice contain thirteen of these substances, which work by blocking HMG-CoA reductase, the enzyme responsible for cholesterol synthesis. The popular "statin" drugs, including Mevacor, work by inhibiting the same enzyme.

Is red yeast rice really safe?

Toxicity studies using rabbits, quails, rats, and mice have all found red yeast rice to be a safe and effective supplement. One study even fed rats the equivalent of 600 times the daily dose for humans and no adverse affects were seen. XueZhiKan, a concentrated extract of red yeast rice, has been shown not to damage either mouse chromosomes or sperm. No serious side effects have been found in any of the human trials.

What kind of side effects were seen?

The side effects seen in the human studies have been mild and mainly gastrointestinal. Researchers in a Chinese study of 446 patients using Cholestin reported: "Although mild side effects (i.e., heartburn, flatulence, and dizziness) were found in a few patients, these symptoms resolved quickly."

In the American study with Cholestin, three subjects in the placebo group reported minor side effects while no side effects were seen in those actually taking the supplement. Manufacturers suggest that you take the supplement on a full stomach to minimize any gastrointestinal discomfort.

Who should take red yeast rice?

Red yeast rice was developed for men and postmenopausal women with moderately elevated cholesterol between 200 and 240 mg/dL. If your cholesterol levels are higher, see your doctor before starting therapy.

Is there anyone who should not take red yeast rice?

Although red yeast rice is very safe, there are certain populations who should not use it.

- Anyone who is still growing should not take red yeast rice since dietary cholesterol is necessary for proper brain and nerve development and growth. This includes pregnant women, women who may become pregnant, women who are breast feeding, and young children.
- Red yeast rice has not been tested for safety in children and adolescents so it should not be used by anyone under the age of twenty.
- Since red yeast rice affects the way your liver works it should not be taken by those who have a liver disease, are at risk for liver disease, have a history of liver disease, or have more than two alcoholic drinks a day.
- Do not take red yeast rice if you have had an organ transplant or major surgery, have a serious infection, disease, or physical disorder.

What is the difference between red yeast rice and lovastatin, the prescription drug?

Red yeast rice is a natural product that contains thirteen different HMG-CoA reductase inhibitors, phytosterols including beta sitosterol, campesterol, stigmasterol, and sapogenin, and a mixture of fatty acids. Lovastatin is a prescription-only drug that contains one isolated purified

HMG-CoA reductase inhibitor. Lovastatin is recommended for individuals with elevated cholesterol levels. Red yeast rice is recommended for those with moderately elevated or border-line cholesterol levels.

Can I take red yeast rice *and* another supplement that lowers cholesterol?

Yes, you can safely combine red yeast rice with most recommended supplements including fish oil (omega-3 fatty acids) commonly recommended for high triacylglyceride levels, folic acid and vitamins B6 and B12 (B complex) supplements recommended for high homocysteine levels, soluble fiber supplements, conjugated linoleic acid and garlic pills recommended for high cholesterol, antioxidant supplements, and the magnesium, calcium and other mineral supplements recommended for high blood pressure.

You cannot combine red yeast rice with another prescribed, cholesterol lowering medicine.

If my cholesterol levels do not decrease, can I take more than the recommended 1.2 grams?

Do not take more red yeast rice without the guidance of a knowledgeable physician. More is not always better.

I don't want to follow a diet, I just want to take the red yeast rice pills. Can I do that?

If you want to experience the results seen in the clinical studies with red yeast rice, you must follow a Step I diet. If you are not the type to follow diets, here are five easy steps that will have much the same effect.

1. Eat more fruits and vegetables, at least seven servings a day. No way around this one. Yes, food supplements are important, but they cannot substitute for real food.

2. Have at least one serving a soy foods a day. A glass of cold soy milk is one easy way.
3. Take a balanced vitamin, mineral, and antioxidant supplement.
4. Greatly decrease the amount of junk food you eat. If you sit down in front of the TV and down a bag of greasy potato chips or a whole package of cookies, find a healthier substitute or break the habit.
5. Stop eating at fast food restaurants. Find some other eatery that you like which serves healthier food, preferably one that serves vegetables.

Do nothing else and you can see dramatic changes in your health. Of course, this diet is not only heart friendly. The enzyme systems that prevent oxidation of your LDL are also the ones that protect you from cancer. Fruits and vegetables also provide the nutrients necessary for strong bones and can help prevent the development of osteoporosis. In fact, research has shown over and over again that a diet rich in fruits and vegetables decreases your risk of developing almost any disease.

Nutrients that Prevent LDL Oxidation

• Vitamin E	• Carotenes	• CoEnzyme Q10
• Vitamin C	• Flavonoids	• Selenium
• Vitamin B6	• Glutathione	

FREQUENTLY ASKED QUESTIONS ABOUT FAT

How much fat can I eat?

Total fat intake should be no more 30 percent of total calories. I don't suggest you limit your fat intake because fat is necessarily bad but because it is a concentrated energy source that, in excess, will contribute to obesity. There are some kinds of fats you should not eat, but good fats are necessary for a healthy body and heart.

Fat here is shown as a percentage of the total number of calories you eat in one day. For example, let's say you eat about 2,000 calories a day. Thirty percent of 2,000 would be 600 calories (0.30 times 2,000). Therefore, you want to get no more than 600 calories a day from fat. Once you have calculated how many calories you consume, look up how many fat grams you can eat during the day from Table 7-1. Instructions for calculating caloric needs can be found in Chapter 8.

Table 7-1:
How Much Fat Is Thirty Percent?

The total number of calories is found in the far left column. Look across to find how many calories from fat and fat grams this translates into.

| | TOTAL FAT | | SATURATED FAT | |
TOTAL CALORIES	FAT CALORIES	FAT GRAMS	SAT CALORIES	SAT GRAMS
1200 calories	360 calories	40 grams	120 calories	14 grams
1400 calories	420 calories	47 grams	140 calories	16 grams
1600 calories	480 calories	53 grams	160 calories	18 grams
1800 calories	540 calories	60 grams	180 calories	20 grams
2000 calories	600 calories	66 grams	200 calories	22 grams
2200 calories	660 calories	72 grams	220 calories	24 grams
2400 calories	720 calories	81 grams	240 calories	27 grams
2600 calories	780 calories	87 grams	260 calories	29 grams
2800 calories	860 calories	93 grams	289 calories	31 grams
3000 calories	920 calories	99 grams	300 calories	33 grams

How much fat is that by weight?

600 calories at 9 calories of fat per gram works out to 66 grams of fat (600 divided by 9) a day. Food labels will tell you how much fat a product contains.

Does this mean I can't eat a food that gets more than 30 percent of its calories from fat?

Very often people misunderstand what 30 percent means. It refers to how much total fat you should eat in any one-day period. It does *not* mean that foods with less than 30 percent calories from fat are good. It does *not* mean that foods with more than 30 percent calories from fat are bad. It does *not* mean that all meals or recipes must be balanced with 30 percent of their calories coming from fat. It only means that *at the end of the day* only 30 percent of your calories came from fat. Some very healthy foods are high in fat. For example, some nuts contain 70 percent calories from fat, but their consumption is linked to a decrease in heart disease. If weight control is an issue, you will want to eat your high-fat meals during the first part of the day. Fat is more likely to be stored when eaten later in the day. A high carbohydrate meal is a good idea in the evening since it promotes the manufacture of serotonin, the sleep neurotransmitter.

How can you reduce the percentage of calories from fat you eat in a day?

Calories/fat = percentage fat from calories

If you want to decrease your percentage (value on the right), you must either increase the left top number (eat more protein and carbohydrate) or decrease the left bottom number (eat less fat).

If you need to lose weight, decrease the bottom number. That is, eat less fat. If you don't need to lose weight (yes, skinny people can also get atherosclerosis) or if your diet leaves you hungry, increase the top. That is, eat more carbohydrates and plant protein. Either way the result is the same and you consume fewer calories from fat.

A perfect way to decrease your calories from fat is to eat more vegetables. These also provide the antioxidants you need to protect your lipoproteins from oxidation.

Should I limit my cholesterol?

Many government guidelines suggest we limit our cholesterol intake to less than 300 milligrams per day. I haven't included such a recommendation here. For one thing, this recommendation is controversial. Most people have no increase in serum cholesterol when they eat cholesterol. Eggs, which are very rich in cholesterol, have been shown to have no effect on the serum lipids of healthy people.

However, a small percentage of the population *will* experience an increase in serum cholesterol from eating dietary cholesterol. These individuals do need to limit their cholesterol. When you see your doctor for your blood test results, ask him if you should decrease you dietary cholesterol. Foods high in cholesterol include organ meats such as brain, sweetbreads, liver, and kidney; eggs including roe, caviar, and chicken and duck eggs; and foods that include egg yolks such as custards.

For the vast majority of people, the real problem with cholesterol is *oxidized* cholesterol, which has been shown to initiate and accelerate atherosclerosis. You must minimize the amount of oxidized cholesterol in your body as much as you can. This can be done in two ways.

- Do not eat oxidized cholesterol. Avoid all foods that contain dried or heat-treated eggs, milk, cheese, and butterfat.

- Reduce the oxidation of cholesterol in your body. You can do this by eating a diet rich in antioxidant fruits and vegetables. I also recommend that you take an antioxidant supplement that contains vitamins E and C.

If the box says "fat-free," does that make it healthier than the same product that contains fat?

No, the idea that "fat-free" equals healthy comes from the idea that fat is bad. Fat is necessary and too much can be fattening, but this does not mean that foods with no fat are good. Fat makes food more satisfying so you can often eat less without feeling deprived. It also helps you to absorb any fat-soluble vitamins in the food. Fat-free foods usually contain just as many calories as the full fatted version. The fat-free version, however, is usually higher in simple carbohydrates. The "fat-free" label proudly displayed on boxes usually just means this product is refined, high in sugar and calories, low in antioxidants, and devoid of fiber. Not what your arteries need!

What type fats should I eat?

As we read in Chapter 2, monounsaturated fatty acids—MUFAs—appear to prevent both cancer and atherosclerosis. Extra virgin olive oil is a good source of monounsaturated fatty acids, plus it contains antioxidants that make it even more heart healthy. The omega-3 fatty acids are also recommended. They help reduce inflammation, which is strongly implicated in plaque formation.

Oils Rich in Oleic Acid

• Olive oil	• Pecan oil	• Avocado oil
• Cashew oil	• Filbert oil	
• Almond oil	• Macadamia oil	

Are there any bad fats?

There is only one kind of fat that many nutritionists considered to be truly bad. It's not cholesterol or saturated fat; both these fats are natural and have their place when eaten in moderation. It's a type of fat called oxidized fat. You can read more about them in Chapter 3. When cholesterol is heated to high temperatures, it is oxidized (an oxygen atom is added). Oxidation changes the structure and therefore the function of the molecule. Oxidized cholesterol can cause new plaque formation or make existing lesions unstable. Avoid any cholesterol-containing foods that are processed at high temperatures; they probably contain "rusty" cholesterol. The worst culprit here is ghee, a product made by heating butter to a high temperature in order to burn off the milk proteins. The result is a tasty oil that does not burn like regular butter. It is also extremely toxic to your arteries.

Cholesterol is not the only lipid that can oxidize. So can vegetable oils high in polyunsaturated fatty acids such as corn oil, soy, and safflower oil. If you eat at fast food restaurants you will notice that they keep using the same oil to cook in time after time. This prolonged heating causes the oils to break down and oxidize. This is particularly true when vegetable oils rich in fragile polyunsaturated fatty acids are used. I have often wondered why fast food restaurants do not use a more stable oil in which to deep fry. They would certainly be doing their patrons' arteries a favor.

FREQUENTLY ASKED QUESTIONS
ABOUT THE DIET

You keep talking about variety. What is variety in foods and how can I get more variety?

Most of the dietary recommendation you read suggest a varied diet. Unfortunately, to many of us a varied diet means six different ways of cooking your favorite food!

To vary your vegetable intake think "mixed."

- Buy frozen mixed vegetables instead of a single type.
- Eat mixed green salads. Instead of buying a head of iceberg lettuce buy romaine; it contains more vitamins and minerals. Then purchase a small bag of baby mixed salad greens to mix into the romaine to add flavor and interest.
- Eat soups that contain a variety of vegetables. Soup is also a tasty way to get your veggies if you dislike them.
- Prepare a fruit cup with mixed fruits.

To vary your grain intake:

- Buy mixed whole grain bread and bread with nuts and seeds. The sandwiches made from these breads are more filling and interesting than those made from blah white bread.
- Have two or three boxes of cereal on hand in case you get bored with what you have. Don't buy the variety packs—they only include high sugar/low fiber cereals.
- Like hot oatmeal? Other grains also make good breakfast fare.
- Add a generous sprinkle of seeds, whole grain croutons, chopped nuts, or chopped dried fruit to your soups, salads, cooked vegetables, or cooked cereals.
- Hate to cook breakfast in the morning? Use your crock pot to slow cook steel-cut oats overnight. Your breakfast will be waiting for you all warm and inviting when you walk into the kitchen the next morning. And don't limit your crock pot to oatmeal.
- Eat brown rice instead of white. It tastes better and contains the heart healthy bran. Other grains to add to your pilaf include quinoa, barley, wild rice, and amaranth.

Use your food steamer or pressure cooker to cook a week's worth of grains. Then:

1. Add honey and dried fruit for a breakfast grain.
2. Toss the cooked grains in salad dressing for a cold lunch salad.
3. Sprinkle in sliced almonds, miso, and green onions, warm, and you have a dinner pilaf.

What about alcohol?
You should only drink moderately while you are on this diet. Moderately in this case is defined as two drinks for men and one drink for women per day. One drink equals: twelve ounces of regular beer, five ounces of wine, or 1½ ounces of distilled spirits (80 proof).

One day I hear coffee is bad for your heart and the next I hear it's OK. Can I drink coffee?
The conflicting reports on coffee turned out to be the result of the different methods used to brew the coffee. Much of the information linking coffee with elevated cholesterol came from Scandinavia where coffee is boiled, and this association was not consistently seen in the West where coffee is often filtered. The two substances that raise cholesterol have been identified as cafestol and kahweol. Cafestol, and to a lesser extent kahweol, raises serum total and LDL cholesterol in humans. They are not removed by decaffeination but can be removed by a paper filter. Filtered, instant, and percolated coffee have low levels of these substances; espresso has moderate; and French press and boiled coffee the highest.

So yes, you can drink coffee but only if it's drip, percolated, or instant.

What kinds of meats should I eat?

You can eat up to six ounces of meat, low-fat cuts of beef, pork, ham, lamb, veal, or skinless poultry, a day. Fatty meats and well-marbled steaks should only be eaten occasionally as treats. This includes fatty bacon, sausage, hot dogs, and chicken fried steak. If you are going to eat a steak at dinner, either cutback on fat during breakfast and lunch or eat a plate full of vegetables with the steak.

- Choose only lean cuts of meat such as round and loin (top round and round tip or sirloin, hamburger with 15 percent fat). Pass on cuts that are marbled.
- Trim all visible fat from the meat. This includes the skin of poultry and the rim of fat around the edge of beef. Trimming can cut the fat content of a piece of meat by 50 percent. You can roast a bird with the skin on to lock in moisture and then remove it before serving.
- Use low-fat cooking methods. Instead of breading and frying, roast, broil, microwave, bake, or stir-fry. When roasting, place the meat on a rack so the fat can drip away. Pressure cooking is an ideal way to prepare tough cuts quickly.
- To remove the fat from soups and stews, first refrigerate and then skim the hardened fat off the top.

Is snacking allowed on this diet?

Baby boomers were taught that the ideal meal pattern was three square meals a day with no snacks to "ruin the appetite." We know now that this was not very ideal at all. These large meals spaced so far apart resulted in long periods of time with no food. This led to blood glucose and insulin levels that went up with meals and down after. Those ups and downs can be detrimental to your health. It is better to eat five to six smaller meals a day. This keeps glucose and the resultant insulin levels more even. High insulin levels can damage the endothelium, and some feel they may be one of the causes of atherosclerosis. Just remember to keep those snacks or small meals healthy. No junk food.

How much is in one serving?

Use the chart below or this "handy" method. Make a fist. This is the size of one cup or two servings of cooked vegetables. Open you hand. Your palm is equal to one serving of meat and it will hold one serving of snack chips or nuts. The length of your index finger is the diameter of one medium serving of fruit. Your thumb volume is about two tablespoons, one serving of nut butter, one ounce or twenty-eight grams, one fluid ounce or 30 ml, or one-half serving of cheese. The tip of your thumb holds about one teaspoon or one serving of oil. Now you will never be without your measuring spoons and cups!

How you perceive a serving depends a lot on the size of your appetite. A person with a large appetite will see one and one-half cups as a one-cup serving, while a person with a small appetite will see one-half cup as a one-cup serving. To avoid this, measure your food for the first day or two. Of course, if you are using the "handy" method, a person with large hands is more likely to need larger portions and the person with smaller hands, smaller portions.

Since variety of food is more important than quantity of the food, decrease your serving size if you want to lose weight or if your appetite and caloric needs are low. If you need to gain weight or if you are still hungry, increase the number of servings.

Bread, Cereal, Potato, and Legumes Group
1 slice of bread
1 ounce of ready-to-eat cereal (1 ounce = 1/4 cup to 2 cups
     depending on cereal)
1/2 cup of cooked dry beans, peas, or lentils
1/2 cup of cooked cereal, rice, potatoes, or pasta
1/2 bun, bagel, or English muffin
3 or 4 plain crackers (small)
1 medium whole potato

Vegetable Group
1 cup of raw leafy vegetables
1/2 cup cooked or chopped raw
1/2 cup fresh vegetable juice
1 medium whole vegetable

Fruit Group
1 medium apple, banana, orange, nectarine, peach
1/2 cup of chopped, cooked, or dried fruit
3/4 cup of fruit juice

Milk, Yogurt, and Cheese Group
1 cup of milk or yogurt
1.5 ounces of natural cheese (a thin slice or one-inch cube)

Poultry, Fish, Eggs, and Nuts and Seeds Group
2 to 3 ounces of cooked poultry or fish (about the size of a
     deck of cards)
1 egg
2 tablespoons of nut butter
Handful of seeds or shelled nuts

Oil, Fat, and Sweets Group
1 teaspoon butter, oil, margarine
2 teaspoons mayonnaise or nut butters
1 tablespoon salad dressing
1 tablespoon cream cheese
2 teaspoons lowfat margarine or spread
3 teaspoons seeds or nuts
1/8 medium avocado
10 small or 5 large olives
1 teaspoon sugar, honey, or other liquid natural sweetener

I am not used to cooking with whole foods. Any tips on how to prepare them?

Treat yourself to some new cookbooks. There a large number of whole food cookbooks available. Buy several to learn some new tricks. This is especially important if you do not like vegetables. Take the time to identify some recipes that will make you look forward to eating your veggies. You might also want to invest in a few new food appliances.

- A juicer is fun to have. If you cannot manage to eat all of the recommended vegetable servings, try juicing some of them. Drink juices with meals for better absorption of nutrients.
- Want to eat more legumes but they take too long to cook? Get yourself a pressure cooker. Beans and whole grains cook in a snap when you use a pressure cooker to prepare them. Those flavorful low-fat cuts of meat also cook up quickly. I use my cooker to make vegetable stew in less than fifteen minutes.
- Get acquainted with rice cookers (also called vegetable steamers). These appliances cost very little but offer great convenience. Grains prepared in them come out fluffy and light. Best of all, the cooking food needs no supervision. The steamer turns itself off so you can never burn

either the steamer or your food. I like to let mine do the cooking while I run errands. Of course these steamers are the best way to cook delicate greens. They never come out mushy or watery.

- Crock pots or slow cookers are another good idea that have never gone out of fashion. I use mine to cook steel-cut oatmeal overnight. In the morning I have only to ladle the porridge into a bowl. It's faster than instant oatmeal and vastly superior in taste and texture. Slow cookers will also cook low-fat cuts of meat while you work.
- Have a microwave oven? You can buy cookware that will turn your microwave into a pressure cooker, slow cooker, or rice steamer.
- Make your own whole grain bread in a bread machine. Prices have really come down so that almost anyone can now afford the luxury of freshly baked bread. Set the bread to bake overnight so that you awake to the aroma of a fresh loaf.

You recommend one serving of soy foods a day. What are soy foods?

Soy food are simply foods made from soy. Soy is just as versatile as milk and much more health promoting. Soybeans can be sprouted, steamed, boiled, fermented, roasted, curdled, or dried. There are so many different types of soy products it is easy to work them into your everyday diet.

- Soybeans mature in the pod into a hard dry bean. Add them to soup and stews just as you would other beans.
- Soybeans can be sprouted or picked when they are still sweet and green (edamame) and eaten as a green vegetable.
- Instead of potato chips when you want a snack, have a handful of soy nuts. Soy nuts are made from whole soybeans that have been soaked and then roasted.

- Soy milk is probably the easiest way to add soy to your diet. This tasty milk-like beverage is made by boiling ground, whole soybeans in water and separating the liquid from the fiber. Soy milk is available in a variety of flavors and types including plain, whole fat, low fat, fat free, fortified, and vanilla and cocoa flavored. Serve it well chilled. I prefer the fresh brands of soy milk found in the dairy case rather than the varieties sold in aseptic containers.

- Tofu is the most common type of soy food found in American grocery stores. It is made by curdling fresh hot soy milk in a process similar to making cottage cheese. Tofu takes on the taste of whatever is added. This can be your favorite dip mix or instant pudding mix. Firm and extra firm tofu are best used in recipes where you want the tofu to hold its shape, for example, in stir fries or grilling. Medium soft tofu works well when you need a softer product for use in puddings, fillings, cheesecakes, and salads. Soft tofu is used in blending to make savory dressings and dips or creamy desserts.

- Just as milk is used to make cheese and yogurt, soy milk is also used to make soy cheese and soy yogurt. Since these products are not made from milk they are lactose- and whey- and casein-free, making them a good choice for those with milk allergies or intolerance.

- Whole soybeans are mixed with rice or millet and then fermented to produce a product called tempeh. Tempeh has a nutty, smoky taste with a mushroom-like aroma. It makes a good meat replacement in recipes.

- Miso is another fermented soy product. It is a made by fermenting a blend of whole soybeans, a grain, salt, and a culture in cedar vats for up to three years. The result is a smooth paste with a fragrant aroma. Use miso to make a broth or use as a seasoning in soups and stews.

- Instant soy protein powder quickly mixes into any liquid. Blend it with strawberries and a banana for a smoothie.

What is fiber and why is it so important?

Fiber is the part of food that resists digestion by human enzymes. It cannot leave the digestive system, yet it still manages to influence metabolism. Insoluble fiber is the type of fiber that does not dissolve in water. It is found in plant cell walls and when eaten absorbs and holds water, increasing the bulk of the feces. Diets rich in insoluble fiber are associated with lower rates of certain types of cancer.

The other type of fiber is soluble fiber, the type that dissolves in water to form a gel. Diets rich in soluble fiber are strongly associated with a lower risk of atherosclerosis, and research has shown that fiber supplements can lower cholesterol levels. The mechanism behind this is not yet understood. Soluble fiber may bind the cholesterol contained in bile so that it cannot be absorbed. This means the liver must use its own cholesterol to replace that lost in the bile, which results in a decrease in total cholesterol. It may also be due to short chain fatty acids (SCFA). When soluble fiber reaches the colon, some of it is digested by the friendly bacteria that grow there and get fermented into SCFA. These fatty acids are not confined to the intestine and can enter circulation where they travel to the liver and in some way decrease cholesterol production.

Which foods can I eat to get soluble fiber?

Soluble fiber can be found in most fruits and vegetables but is richest in citrus fruits, apples, pears, barley, brown rice, oatmeal and oat cereals, and most especially in oat bran, rice bran, ground flaxseed, and psyllium seed. The latter two *must* be mixed with a liquid before consuming them. You can buy soluble fiber supplements, but soluble fiber-rich foods also contain antioxidants that will protect your LDL from oxidation. There are only two fiber supplements that have been tested for effectiveness: Shaklee's Fiber Plan from Shaklee Corporation, which is a mixture of the soluble fibers psyllium, pectin, guar gum, and locust bean gum, and Metamucil made by Procter & Gamble, which contains the soluble fiber psyllium. Both must be mixed with a liquid; do not attempt to eat them dry.

FREQUENTLY ASKED QUESTIONS ABOUT VITAMINS AND MINERALS

What are antioxidants and which foods contain them?

Antioxidants are substances that stop oxidation and free radical damage. They help to protect your endothelial cells and LDL particles from the damage that initiates atherosclerosis. The major antioxidants are vitamins C and E and the carotenes and flavonoids. Selenium, zinc, and copper are necessary parts of the body's antioxidant enzyme systems.

Fruits, vegetables, and whole grains are all such excellent sources of antioxidants it's impossible to single out just a few. It's one of the reasons they are recommended so often by nutrition experts and why they are such an important part of this diet. Although you can take antioxidant supplements, they are probably not as effective as those found in real food. There is no substitute for real food.

Sources of Vitamin C

- Broccoli
- Cabbage
- Cantaloupe
- Citrus fruits
- Collard greens
- Kale
- Mangos
- Papaya
- Strawberries
- Sweet peppers
- Turnip greens

Sources of Vitamin E

- Nuts
- Wheat germ oil

Do I have to drink milk to get my calcium?

No, but milk is a convenient source of calcium and protein. If you do not drink milk, drink calcium-enriched orange juice or soy milk, calcium-rich foods (see Table 7-2), or take a calcium supplement.

Table 7-2: Calcium-Rich Foods

Almonds	1 ounce	80 mg
Blackstrap molasses	1 tablespoon	172 mg
Broccoli	1/2 cup	88 mg
Collards	1/2 cup	152 mg
Dandelion greens	1/2 cup	73 mg
Edamame	1/2 cup	130 mg
Figs, dried	10 figs	269 mg
Kale	1/2 cup	134 mg
Milk	1/2 cup	151 mg
Mustard greens	1/2 cup	183 mg
OJ, calcium fortified	1/2 cup	150 mg
Okra	1/2 cup	92 mg
Perch	3 oz	117 mg
Pike	3 oz	120 mg
Salmon with bones	3 oz	200 mg
Soybean nuts, roasted	1/2 cup	119 mg
Tahini	1 ounce	64 mg
Tempeh	1/2 cup	77 mg
Tofu, firm	1/2 cup	258 mg
Turnip greens	1/2 cup	75 mg
Yogurt	1/2 cup	207 mg

What other minerals can help prevent heart disease?

- *Magnesium.* Scientists have noted that Greenlanders have diets rich in magnesium with a low incidence of ischemic heart disease and hypertension. Danes, on the other hand, eat diets high in processed foods and low in magnesium with a high incidence of IHD and hypertension. When Greenlanders move to Denmark they eventually acquire the same incidence for these diseases as the indigenous Danes. Could it be the magnesium? Magnesium can lower blood pressure, relieve angina, prevent calcium deposits in plaque, and cause the muscles of the arteries to relax.

- *Calcium*. Calcium works with magnesium to regulate the heartbeat. It has also been shown to decrease blood pressure which contributes to atherosclerosis.

- *Potassium*. Like calcium, potassium is involved in the regulation of blood pressure. Populations with low levels of dietary potassium have a high incidence of hypertension. Hypertension is a well-recognized risk factor for atherosclerosis.

- *Selenium*. This mineral is an important part of the antioxidant enzyme glutathione peroxidase. There is an association between the selenium content of the soil and that area's risk of atherosclerosis. The so-called "stroke belt" of the United States (includes part of Georgia and the Carolinas) has a very low level of selenium in the soil while having a very high incidence of heart disease. Do not supplement with more than 200 micrograms of selenium.

- *Zinc*. Zinc is a part of the antioxidant enzyme superoxide dismutase. It may help to reduce total cholesterol and LDL, and increase HDL. When your zinc levels are low you need more vitamin E.

- *Copper*. This mineral is part of two antioxidant enzymes: superoxide dismutase and ceruloplasmin. A copper deficiency, according to research, makes your LDL more susceptible to oxidation.

Food sources of calcium, magnesium, potassium, zinc, selenium, and copper can be found in Tables 7-2 through 7-7. If you take a calcium or magnesium supplement, I recommend either a citrate or malate form (for example, calcium citrate or malate and magnesium citrate or malate). These forms are not only well-absorbed but may help to prevent calcium loss in the urine by keeping your blood more alkaline.

Table 7-3: Magnesium-Rich Foods

Almonds	1 ounce	86 mg
Avocado	1 medium	90 mg
Baked potato	1 medium	55 mg
Bean sprouts	3 ounces	111 mg
Cashews	1 ounce	74 mg
Chickpeas	1 cup	78 mg
Dock	1/2 cup	69 mg
Dried beans, cooked	1 cup	100 mg
Figs, dried	10 figs	111 mg
Filberts	1 ounce	84 mg
Lentils	1 cup	71 mg
Mackerel, Atlantic	3 ounces	83 mg
Oat bran	1/2 cup	44 mg
Oysters	1 dozen	92 mg
Pumpkin seeds	1 ounce	152 mg
Rice bran	1 ounce	219 mg
Sesame seeds	1 ounce	101 mg
Soybean nuts	1/2 cup	196 mg
Soybeans	1 cup	148 mg
Split peas	1 cup	71 mg
Sun-dried tomatoes	1/2 cup	52 mg
Sunflower seeds	1 ounce	100 mg
Tempeh	1/2 cup	58 mg
Tofu, firm	1/2 cup	118 mg

Tomato paste	1/2 cup	67 mg
Watermelon seeds	1 ounce	146 mg
Wheat germ/bran	1/4 cup	75 mg

Table 7-4: Potassium-Rich Foods

Apricots, dried	10 rings	482 mg
Avocado	1 medium	1200 mg
Bamboo shoots	1/2 cup	405 mg
Banana	1 medium	451 mg
Beans	1 cup	950 mg
Blackstrap molasses	1 tablespoon	498 mg
Cantaloupe	1 cup	494 mg
Dates, dried	10 dates	541 mg
Figs, dried	10 dates	1332 mg
Honeydew melon	1 cup	461 mg
Milk, skim	1 cup	406 mg
Papaya	1 medium	780 mg
Potato, baked	1 medium	844 mg
Prune juice	1 cup	706 mg
Prunes	10 prunes	626 mg
Raisins	2/3 cup	825 mg
Soybean nuts	1/2 cup	1200 mg
Sun-dried tomatoes	1/2 cup	925 mg
Tomato paste	1/2 cup	1221 mg
Yogurt	1 cup	590 mg

Table 7-5: Sources of Zinc

Almonds	Lima beans	Soy lecithin
Anchovies	Nuts	Split peas
Egg yolk	Potatoes	Turnips
Garlic	Sardines	Walnut
Haddock	Shellfish	Whole grains

Table 7-6: Sources of Selenium

Barley	Lobster	Shrimp
Brazil nuts	Oysters	Sunflower seeds
Brown rice	Red Swiss chard	Swordfish
Haddock	Salmon	Tuna

Table 7-7: Sources of Copper

Legumes	Nuts	Shellfish

You have mentioned a vitamin supplement, but there are so many. How do you choose a good one?

You should take three types of food supplements. Very often supplement types are mixed. For example, I take a formula that is a combined vitamin/mineral supplement. My son takes a formula that is a combined vitamin/antioxidant formula. It is important that you read labels when combining food supplements so that you do not get too much of a fat-soluble vitamin or trace mineral (selenium can be toxic at levels above 800 mcg).

1. A vitamin supplement that contains all the fat- and water-soluble vitamins.

2. A mineral supplement that includes calcium, magnesium, zinc, copper, chromium, and selenium. Do not take a formula that contains iron (too much iron is associated with atherosclerosis).

3. An antioxidant supplement. It should contain a wide variety of antioxidants including vitamin C, selenium (if not included in the mineral supplement), mixed carotenes (including beta carotene—no more than 10,000 units—and lycopene), and mixed tocopherols with at least 400 IU of vitamin E. Look for a formula that includes some of these additional antioxidants: coenzyme Q10, lipoic acid, rosemary extract, green tea extract, and flavonoids such as proanthocyanidins (grape seed and pine bark extract).

- Look for a comprehensive, balanced food supplement. That is, a formula that contains a little of a lot. It should have 100 percent of the RDA, not 1,000 percent. Some manufacturers stick a lot of the cheaper vitamins into the tablet to impress you but then skimp on the important more expensive ones.

- Look for tablets that will dissolve easily and are easy for you to swallow. If you cannot swallow tablets, vitamins are available as powders, chewables, or liquid.

- You should also take a coenzyme Q10 supplement. The enzyme HMG-CoA reductase is necessary for the manufacture of CoQ10, so its levels are lowered by the HMG-CoA reductase inhibitors found in red yeast rice. CoQ10 is an enzyme that is necessary for energy production. It also works as an antioxidant by recycling vitamin E and helps to prevent the production of homocysteine, which can damage arterial walls.

Sources of CoQ10

- Fish
- Meats
- Rapeseed oils
- Rice bran
- Sesame seed oil
- Soy and some other legumes
- Soybean oil
- Wheat germ

I have heard that some of the B vitamins can prevent atherosclerosis. Is this true?

Yes. Adequate levels of pyridoxine (B6), vitamin B12, and folate can prevent a condition called homocysteinemia, or high levels of homocysteine.

Homocysteine is a naturally occurring substance produced during amino acid metabolism. Homocysteine is broken down into taurine, which requires vitamin B6, or is recycled back into methionine, which requires vitamin B12 and folate. If not enough of these B complex vitamins are available, homocysteine levels can rise. This is of interest to us because a high level of homocysteine is toxic to endothelial cells and promotes the oxidation of LDL particles. Even a moderate elevation of homocysteine is an important risk factor for premature cardiovascular disease.

By consuming enough pyridoxine (B6), vitamin B12, and folate, you can reduce your serum levels of homocysteine and slow the progress of atherosclerosis and decrease your chance of developing other types of cardiovascular disease. See the sidebars for foods rich in these nutrients.

Sources of Vitamin B12
- Fish
- Milk
- Skinless poultry
- Yogurt

Sources of Folacin
- Almonds
- Asparagus
- Barley
- Beans
- Black-eyed peas
- Brewer's yeast
- Green cruciferous vegetables
- Leafy green vegetables
- Lentils
- Oatmeal
- Soy foods
- Split peas
- Walnuts
- Wheat and rice germ and bran
- Whole wheat

Sources of Vitamin B6
- Avocados
- Bananas
- Beans
- Brewer's yeast
- Brown rice
- Halibut
- Hazelnuts
- Kale
- Mackerel
- Salmon
- Sunflower seeds
- Trout
- Tuna fish
- Walnuts
- Wheat germ

8

Charting Your Progress

We are getting near the end of the book, and it's time to put all the knowledge you have gained to work. You now understand about lipoproteins and how they can affect your body. You know what red yeast rice is and what it can do for you. You have read the red yeast diet and know how to follow it. Now it is time to talk about *you*. What are *your* test results? What are *your* risks? What are *your* goals?

The first part of this chapter is a convenient place to record all your test results and list your goals. Just read and follow the instructions for each set of forms. The second part of the chapter will help you to understand what all those numbers mean. The last part will help you to calculate your own risk of developing cardiovascular disease.

If you haven't done so yet, now is the time to have your blood cholesterol levels tested. You should also evaluate your diet to see what areas need improvement. The presence of other risk factors will change how your doctor views your cholesterol level, so be sure to do the risk evaluation.

As you read through this chapter, fill in the blanks and then record the information. This way you will be able to see at a glance areas in which you have made progress and those that need improvement.

LIPID AND BLOOD PRESSURE EVALUATION

Instructions

1. Record your cholesterol levels as milligrams per deciliter (mg/dl) of blood and then read the section "How to Understand Your Cholesterol Test Results." See the sidebar for instructions on converting test numbers given in millimoles to deciliters.

2. Together with your physician, determine your lipid level goals. Recommended levels can be found in Table 8-1.

Table 8-1: Cholesterol Levels

TOTAL CHOLESTEROL	DESIRABLE BELOW 200	BORDERLINE 200–240	UNDESIRABLE ABOVE 240
HDL	Above 45	35–45	Below 35
Triglycerides	Below 200	200–400	Above 400
LDL	Below 130	130–160	Above 160
Total /HDL	Below 4.5	4.5–5.5	Above 5.5
LDL/HDL	Below 3	3–5	Above 5

3. Record your blood pressure and read the section "How to Understand Your Blood Pressure Readings."

How to Convert Millimoles per Liter into to Milligrams per Liter

Help! My cholesterol numbers don't make sense. Instead of being in the hundreds, they are in single digits. What's wrong?

In the United States, cholesterol and triglycerides are usually measured in milligrams per deciliter of blood (mg/dL). A deciliter is one-tenth of a liter. In some countries cholesterol is measured in millimoles per liter. If your results are small numbers under ten, they are probably given in millimoles per liter. In order to use these charts you will need to convert your results. Get out the calculator!

To convert cholesterol in millimoles per liter (mmol/L) to milligrams per deciliter (mg/dL), multiply your cholesterol number by 0.01129

$$0.01129 \times mmol/L = mg/dL$$

To convert triglycerides in millimoles per liter (mmol/L) to milligrams per deciliter (mg/dL), multiply your triglyceride number by 0.02586

$$0.02586 \times mmol/L = mg/dL$$

MY TEST RESULTS:

Base test date: _____

	Total Blood				
	Cholesterol	LDL	HDL	TAG	Pressure
Actual :	_____	_____	_____	_____	_____
Goal :	_____	_____	_____	_____	_____

Follow-up 1 test date: _____

	Total Blood				
	Cholesterol	LDL	HDL	TAG	Pressure
Actual :	_____	_____	_____	_____	_____
Goal :	_____	_____	_____	_____	_____

Follow-up 2 test date: _____

	Total Blood				
	Cholesterol	LDL	HDL	TAG	Pressure
Actual :	_____	_____	_____	_____	_____
Goal :	_____	_____	_____	_____	_____

Follow-up 3 test date: _____

	Total Blood				
	Cholesterol	LDL	HDL	TAG	Pressure
Actual :	_____	_____	_____	_____	_____
Goal :	_____	_____	_____	_____	_____

Follow-up 4 test date: _____

	Total Blood				
	Cholesterol	LDL	HDL	TAG	Pressure
Actual :	_____	_____	_____	_____	_____
Goal :	_____	_____	_____	_____	_____

WEIGHT EVALUATION

Instructions

1. Weigh yourself in the morning without clothes and fill in this number. Always weigh yourself at the same time as your weight will vary during the day.
2. Have a friend measure your height stretching yourself as tall as you can. Do this in the morning since you will lose height during the day.
3. Your goal weight should be realistic. It is not necessary to reduce your weight to that recommended by the weight-height tables.
4. Calculate your BMI (body mass index). Instructions for calculating this number can be found later in the chapter. It can help you determine whether you are overweight.
5. Calculate your IBW (ideal body weight). Instructions for calculating this number can be found later in the chapter. It can also help you determine whether you are overweight.

How to calculate your waist-to-hip ratio:

- With a measuring tape measure around your waist near your navel while you stand relaxed. Do not pull in your stomach.
- Measure your hips where they are largest, over the buttocks.

- Divide the waist measure by the hips measure to get your waist-to-hip ratio.

    A waist-to-hip ratio of greater than 0.9 in men and 0.8 in women is defined as an apple shape.

What is your waist-to-hip ratio? _____
Are you an apple or a pear? _____

MY TEST RESULTS:

Base test date: _____

	Weight	Height	BMI	IBW
Actual :	_____	_____	_____	_____
Goal :	_____	_____	_____	_____

Follow-up 1 test date: _____

	Weight	Height	BMI	IBW
Actual :	_____	_____	_____	_____
Goal :	_____	_____	_____	_____

Follow-up 2 test date: _____

	Weight	Height	BMI	IBW
Actual :	_____	_____	_____	_____
Goal :	_____	_____	_____	_____

Follow-up 3 test date: _____

	Weight	Height	BMI	IBW
Actual :	_____	_____	_____	_____
Goal :	_____	_____	_____	_____

Follow-up 4 test date: _____

	Weight	Height	BMI	IBW
Actual :	_____	_____	_____	_____
Goal :	_____	_____	_____	_____

DIET EVALUATION

Instructions

1. Read Chapter 7 and record your food group intake below.
2. Record your goal (recommended) intake. If you have a low calorie intake or are trying to lose weight, choose the lower amount of recommended servings. If you have a large calorie intake or are trying to gain weight, choose the higher amount of recommended servings.
3. Calculate your caloric needs and record the number. Instruction can be found in the section "How Many Calories Do You Need?"
4. Look up your caloric intake in Table 8-2 to determine the amounts of total fat and saturated fat you should be consuming.

Table 8-2: Recommended Fat and Saturated Fat Intake for the Red Yeast Rice Diet

Round off the number of calories you eat each day and locate that number on the right. To the left of the number you will find the number of total and saturated fat calories and fat grams you can eat each day.

	TOTAL FAT		SATURATED FAT	
Total calories	Fat calories	Fat grams	Sat Calories	Sat Grams
1200 calories	360 calories	40 grams	120 calories	14 grams
1400 calories	420 calories	47 grams	140 calories	16 grams
1600 calories	480 calories	53 grams	160 calories	18 grams
1800 calories	540 calories	60 grams	180 calories	20 grams
2000 calories	600 calories	66 grams	200 calories	22 grams
2200 calories	660 calories	73 grams	220 calories	24 grams
2400 calories	720 calories	80 grams	240 calories	27 grams
2600 calories	780 calories	86 grams	260 calories	29 grams
2800 calories	840 calories	93 grams	289 calories	31 grams
3000 calories	900 calories	100 grams	300 calories	33 grams
3200 calories	960 calories	106 grams	300 calories	33 grams
3400 calories	1020 calories	113 grams	300 calories	33 grams
3600 calories	1080 calories	120 grams	300 calories	33 grams
3800 calories	1140 calories	126 grams	300 calories	33 grams
4000 calories	1200 calories	133 grams	300 calories	33 grams
4200 calories	1260 calories	139 grams	300 calories	33 grams
4400 calories	1320 calories	146 grams	300 calories	33 grams
4600 calories	1380 calories	153 grams	300 calories	33 grams
4800 calories	1440 calories	159 grams	300 calories	33 grams
5000 calories	1500 calories	166 grams	300 calories	33 grams

NUMBER OF SERVINGS
(FOR SERVING SIZE SEE CHAPTER 7)

PRESENT INTAKE	YOUR GOAL	FOLLOW-UP 1	FOLLOW-UP 2	FOLLOW-UP 3	FOLLOW-UP 4

Cereals, grains, beans, and potatoes:

_____   _____   _____   _____   _____   _____

Vegetables:

_____   _____   _____   _____   _____   _____

Fruits:

_____   _____   _____   _____   _____   _____

Dairy:

_____   _____   _____   _____   _____   _____

Soy:

_____   _____   _____   _____   _____   _____

Meats, fish, and eggs:

_____   _____   _____   _____   _____   _____

Oil, fats, and sweets:

_____   _____   _____   _____   _____   _____

Water:

_____   _____   _____   _____   _____   _____

PRESENT INTAKE	YOUR GOAL	FOLLOW-UP 1	FOLLOW-UP 2	FOLLOW-UP 3	FOLLOW-UP 4

Cholesterol-rich foods:

_____ _____ _____ _____ _____ _____

Saturated fat foods:

_____ _____ _____ _____ _____ _____

Junk food:

_____ _____ _____ _____ _____ _____

Vitamin supplement:

_____ _____ _____ _____ _____ _____

Mineral supplement:

_____ _____ _____ _____ _____ _____

Antioxidant supplement:

_____ _____ _____ _____ _____ _____

Number of calories I need each day: _____

Amount of fat I can eat each day: _____

Amount of saturated fat I can eat each day: _____

RISK FACTOR EVALUATION

Instructions

Answer yes or no to each of the questions, then add up the number of yes's. The more you have, the greater your chance of developing cardiovascular disease. If one of your risk factors is high cholesterol, your risk of cardiovascular disease is even greater. For the significance of this number read the section called "What Are Risk Factors?"

	Yes	No
Do you smoke?	_____	_____
Do you have hypertension?	_____	_____
Do you have diabetes?	_____	_____
Are you overweight by 30 percent?	_____	_____
Do you have a sedentary lifestyle?	_____	_____

Hyperlipidemia
Is your total cholesterol high,
    LDL high, or HDL low?   _____   _____

Gender
Are you a man 45 years or older or
    a woman 55 years or older?   _____   _____

Family history of early heart disease
(heart attack or sudden death)
Father or brother stricken before age 55   _____   _____
    or mother or sister stricken before age 65

Total number of risk factors: _____

HOW TO UNDERSTAND YOUR CHOLESTEROL TEST RESULTS

This is the area where the Red Yeast Rice Diet has its greatest impact. You should see a reduction in total cholesterol, LDL cholesterol, and triglycerides and an increase in HDL within eight weeks of starting treatment.

There are two types of cholesterol tests: screening tests and lab tests. Cholesterol screening tests are becoming more common. These are the finger stick tests often done in shopping malls and health fairs. Since these tests are not that accurate and do not measure HDL and LDL, you will need to have more complete testing done at a lab.

Standard cholesterol testing is done in a lab by drawing several tubes of blood. If you have had these blood tests done recently, contact your physician's office for a copy of the results and then fill them in here. Your blood test should measure at least your total cholesterol, HDL cholesterol, and triglycerides. LDL and triglyceride tests might also be performed but involve fasting nine to twelve hours before having your blood drawn.

TOTAL CHOLESTEROL

Total cholesterol is made up of your LDL, HDL, and other blood cholesterol particles. Normal cholesterol is the level at which atherogenesis does not occur, considering other risk factors. Animal and population studies suggest that this is about 160 mg/dL. In the famed Framingham Heart Study, those who had a cholesterol lever lower than 160 mg/dL suffered no heart attacks no matter what their HDL, LDL, or triglyceride levels were. If your total cholesterol level is between 200 and 240 mg/dL, you are a good candidate for treatment with red yeast rice.

LDL

The LDL reading measures your level of LDL cholesterol. This is the cholesterol contained in the LDL particle, which is vulnerable to oxidation. Oxidized LDL particles deposit cholesterol in your arteries. The lower this number is the better. Some laboratories measure LDL directly as part of the blood test. However, some doctors calculate your LDL levels using the following formula:

Total cholesterol—(HDL + [triglycerides/5]) = LDL

HDL

The HDL reading measures your level of HDL cholesterol, the cholesterol contained in the HDL particle that removes cholesterol from your arteries. The higher this number is the better. Research shows that even those with desirable total cholesterol levels are at greater risk if their HDL levels are low. An HDL level below 35 mg/dL puts you at risk of heart disease.

TRIGLYCERIDES

The triglycerides or TG (also called tri*acyl*glycerides or TAG) reading measures the fat in your blood that is being distributed to your tissues. High triglyceride levels are associated with cardiovascular disease. If your triglycerides are between 200 and 400 mg/dL, you are a good candidate for red yeast rice therapy. TAGs must be measured after an overnight fast or the test will pick up triglycerides absorbed from a meal.

RATIOS

In addition to your LDL level, your doctor might calculate the ratios between your total cholesterol and HDL. As the "helpful" HDL levels increase, the ratio decreases, and as HDL decreases the ratio increases. As "bad" LDL levels decrease the ratio decreases, and as the LDL levels increase the ratio increases. The goal is to keep the ratio below 5:1 with the optimum ratio of 3.5:1.

- If a person has a total cholesterol of 200 mg/dL and an HDL cholesterol level of 50 mg/dL, the ratio would be stated as 4:1.
- If the HDL level *decreased* to 40 mg/dL, the ratio would now be 200 to 40 or 5:1. This increase of 10 mg/dL of HDL has unfavorably increased the ratio (and the risk) from 4:1 to 5:1.
- Now if that same person's total cholesterol increased to 240, his ratio would now be 240/40 or 6:1.

While ratios can be helpful, they cannot substitute for knowledge of the actual numbers.

WEIGHT, IBW, AND BMI

There is no single standard definition of obesity and no single best method of measuring the appropriateness of a given weight. Height-weight tables try to indicate the weight ranges at which people of various heights and builds will live the longest. However, we all are aware that weight alone is a poor reflection of body composition. A person can be judged as a healthy weight while having too much fat and too little lean muscle mass. Another person can be judged as overweight while having very little fat and much muscle. Overweight does not necessarily mean over fat. There are two ways to classify obesity. One uses the ideal body weight or IBW and the other uses body mass index or BMI.

How to Calculate Your BMI

It's easy to calculate your Body Mass Index.

BMI = Weight in kilograms/height in meters squared.

If you are not using the metric system, get out your calculator.

1. Multiply your weight in pounds by 0.45. This is your weight in kilograms. For example, if you weigh 150: 150 x 0.45 = 68
2. Multiply your height in inches by 0.025. This is your height in meters. For example, if you're 5'6" (66 inches): 66 x 0.025 = 1.65
3. Square the answer from step 2. (1.65 x 1.65 = 2.72)
4. Divide the answer from step 1 by the answer from step 3. (68/2.72 = 25)

How to Determine if You Are Obese Using BMI

Your BMI should fall within the healthy range of 19 to 25. If you're at the upper end of this range or score more than 25, consider losing enough weight to lower your BMI at least one or two numbers. A BMI of more than 27 is considered overweight. This does not mean you have to diet down to the ideal body weight found in the weight-height tables. Research has shown that you can greatly benefit from a loss of just 20 percent. This means if you are a woman 5'7" who weighs 220 pounds, you will greatly benefit from dieting down to 176 pounds. You don't have to starve yourself to reach your ideal body weight of 135 pounds. This is particularly important if you are an apple shape.

A study published in the May 29, 1998, issue of the journal *Science* found that 54 percent of all U.S. adults are overweight—an increase of about 33 percent since 1978.

Table 8-3: Classification of Obesity Using BMI

BMI RANGE	GRADE
25–29.9	I
30–40	II
> 40	III

HOW TO CALCULATE YOUR IBW

Ideal body weight is far from ideal, but it can be useful.

IBW for men = 110 lb. + 5 lb./inch > 5 feet (+ or − 10 percent)
IBW for women = 100 lb. + 5lb./inch > 5 feet (+ or − 10 percent)

Add 110 pounds for the first 5 feet and then add 5 pounds for each inch above that. For a large frame you add 10 percent. For a small frame subtract 10 percent.

For example, let's say you are a man who is 5'8" tall and have a large frame. To 110 you would add 5 pounds times 8 inches or 110 + (5 x 8) = 150. Add 10 percent (15) for a total of 165 pounds.

Now lets calculate the IBW for a woman who is 5'8" and has a small frame. To 100 you would add 5 pounds times 8 inches or 100 + (5 x 8) = 140. Subtract 10 percent (14) for a total of 126 pounds.

HOW TO DETERMINE IF YOU ARE OBESE USING IBW

To determine if you are obese use this formula:

(Actual weight − IBW) x 100/ IBW

If the man in the first example weighs 220 pounds, we would plug these numbers into the calculation:

(220 − 165) x 100/165 = 33 percent

He is 33 percent overweight, which is categorized as mild obesity. About 90 percent of all overweight persons fall within this mild category.

Based on new evidence and increasing prevalence of obesity, the American Heart Association (AHA) has upgraded obesity to a "major risk factor." The announcement was made at an AHA press conference in New York City and in an article published in the June 2, 1998, issue of the journal *Circulation*. The new categorization by the AHA places obesity in the same group of risk factors as smoking, high blood pressure, high blood cholesterol, and sedentary lifestyle—all factors that people can control to reduce the risk of death and disability from cardiovascular disease.

Table 8-4: Classification of Obesity

PERCENTAGE OVERWEIGHT	OBESITY TYPE
28–40	Mild
41–100	Moderate
>100	Severe

APPLES VERSUS PEARS

Fat is not evenly distributed around the body; it is stored in different patterns. Men usually store their fat deep in the abdomen (the android or apple shape) while women usually store their fat in their hips, thighs, and upper arms (the gynecoid or pear shape). Researchers have discovered that "apples" are at greater risk for heart disease and insulin resistance than "pears."

People with syndrome X (which is explained in the next chapter) are at greater risk for developing cardiovascular disease. It is not the amount of fat a person carries that is related to syndrome X, it is the pattern in which the fat is stored. You do not have to be overweight to fit this pattern. The fat found in "apples" does not specifically cause high cholesterol levels. It is associated with an increase in an apoprotein called apo-B, which is associated with heart disease and is present in those with syndrome X.

Obesity on its own also decreases the number of insulin receptors found on cells so that the normal insulin levels are not enough to do the job. Even a moderate weight loss of 10 to 20 percent can increase the number of receptors to normal levels. One out of every four men over the age of forty have too much abdominal fat and insulin resistance. Women are at greater risk of accumulating visceral fat after menopause.

If you have no other medical problems that will respond to weight loss and if your BMI is between 19 and 25 and your waist-to-hip ratio is less than 0.9 in men and 0.8 in women, then there is no need to lose more weight.

HOW TO UNDERSTAND YOUR BLOOD PRESSURE NUMBERS

Elevated blood pressure or hypertension is a risk factor for cardiovascular disease. You will find a more thorough discussion of this condition in the next chapter.

Your blood pressure is stated as two numbers. For example, let's say that your blood pressure is 110/70 mmHg, which is read as one hundred and ten over seventy millimeters of mercury. This means that the pressure inside the blood vessel being measured is strong enough to force a column of mercury up to a level of 70. The first number, 110, is the *systolic* pressure. This is the pressure taken when the ventricles of the heart are pushing blood into the arteries. The second number, seventy, is the *diastolic* pressure. This is the pressure taken when the ventricles are relaxed. The diastolic pressure is the least pressure that is exerted on the arterial walls. It is the most useful in assessing an individual's risk for heart disease or stroke.

Hypertension occurs when either one or both of these numbers is out of range. *All* elevated readings, whether systolic or diastolic, should receive prompt attention.

Table 8-5: Blood Pressure Ranges

	SYSTOLIC BP	DIASTOLIC BP
Borderline	138–146 mm Hg	84–89 mm Hg
Mild	147–159 mm Hg	90–104 mm Hg
Moderate	160–180 mm Hg	105–114 mm Hg
Severe	> 180 mm Hg	> 114 mm Hg

Let your physician know if someone else in your family has high blood pressure. Hypertension often runs in families, and you may be at greater risk.

Your blood pressure should be checked when you are rested and relaxed. The tension of just being in the doctor's office can sometimes elevate blood pressure. This phenomenon is called white coat hypertension. One blood pressure reading does not mean much. Several checks should be made to get a true average. The cuff should wrap comfortably around your arm since cuffs that are too small or too large will produce false readings.

If you are diagnosed with hypertension, make sure to follow your physician's instructions. Have your pressures checked every two to three months, and if medicine is prescribed, take it as prescribed and continue even after your pressures return to normal.

CALCULATING YOUR CALORIE, FAT, AND SATURATED FAT INTAKE

The Red Yeast Rice Diet is a low-fat diet. To figure out how many fat grams you can eat each day it is necessary to find out how many calories you are now eating. You can do this by keeping a three-day food diary and counting how many calories you eat each day. A faster and easier way is to perform the following calculation:

Daily Calorie Requirement
(for sedentary women) = ____ pounds x 12 = ____ calories

Daily Calorie Requirement
(for sedentary men) = ____ pounds x 14 = ____ calories

Daily Calorie Requirement
(for moderately active women) = ____ pounds x 15 = ____ calories

Daily Calorie Requirement
(for moderately active men) = ____ pounds x 17 = ____ calories

Daily Calorie Requirement
(for active women) = ____ pounds x 18 = ____ calories

Daily Calorie Requirement
(for active men) = ____ pounds x 20 = ____ calories

If you need to lose weight, subtract that amount from your weight before performing the calculations. If you need to gain weight, add it to your weight. For example, a man who weighs 220 pounds has been advised by his doctor to lose twenty pounds. The weight he uses in the calculation is then 200 pounds (220 – 20). This man then needs to eat 3,600 calories (200 times 18) a day. He locates this on the fat chart and discovers he should eat no more than 1,080 grams of total fat or 120 grams of saturated fat.

WHAT ARE RISK FACTORS?

Risk factors are situations that increase your chances of developing cardiovascular disease. Major risk factors are those that medical research has shown to be definitely associated with a significant increase in the risk of cardiovascular disease. They are divided into two groups: those you can change and those you can't.

THOSE YOU CANNOT CHANGE

- *Gender.* Men have a greater risk of heart attack than women, and these attacks happen at an earlier age. Even after menopause, when women's death rate from heart disease increases, it is not as great as men's.
- *Age.* LDL levels rise as you age. Men usually have higher total cholesterol levels than women until they reach forty-five. Up to about this age women also tend to have higher HDL levels then men. After menopause a woman's total cholesterol increases and the protective HDL decreases unless she takes hormone replacement therapy.
- *Family history.* If a close member of your family has elevated lipid levels or other cardiovascular problems, your risk of developing these problems yourself are increased. Likewise, African Americans have more severe hypertension than whites so their risk of cardiovascular disease is greater.

THOSE YOU CAN CONTROL

- *Tobacco use.* Smoking cigarettes damages the walls of your blood vessels, making them prone to injury and plaque formation. Smoking can also lower your HDL by as much as 15 percent! Smoking alone doubles your heart attack risk and is the biggest risk factor for sudden cardiac death. Even involuntary smoking (secondhand smoke) appears to increase the risk of heart disease.

- *Obesity*. As your weight increases, so do your triglycerides. Excess weight can also decrease your HDL. Obesity also influences a number of other risk factors such as blood pressure, blood cholesterol, and triglyceride levels, and makes diabetes more likely to develop. You only have to lose a moderate amount of weight to reduce this risk factor.
- *Diabetes*. Diabetes is notorious for accelerating the development of atherosclerosis. It increases triglycerides and decreases HDL in many people. Diabetes is not always a risk factor you can change and medication may be necessary to control it. If you have diabetes, have yearly blood tests.
- *Hypertension*. By damaging the walls of your arteries, high blood pressure can accelerate the development of atherosclerosis. Be aware that some medications for high blood pressure can increase LDL and triglyceride levels and decrease HDL levels. Make sure you have your lipid levels checked yearly.
- *Inactivity*. A sedentary lifestyle is well associated with a decrease in HDL. While aerobic exercise is one way to increase your HDL, even thirty to forty-five minutes of brisk walking every other day helps protect your cardiovascular system.

LET YOUR DOCTOR KNOW

Now that you have identified your risk factors, what do you do with them? Once you know your weak spots, you can set goals to change them. They should also serve as motivation to follow the Red Yeast Rice Diet. It also does you no good to keep your risk factors to yourself. Make sure your physician knows all of them and that they are recorded in your medical records. *The presence of other risk factors will change how your doctor views your cholesterol levels.*

Risk factors are interrelated. For example, let's say you are sedentary. Exercise will help you to lose weight, which will help you decrease your blood pressure and improve your insulin tolerance. It will also reduce your "bad" cholesterol levels and increase your "good." When you eliminate one risk you reduce or eliminate others. Each risk factor may also influence your lipid levels.

The more risk factors you have, in combination with undesirable lipid levels, the greater your risk of developing cardiovascular disease. If you have several risk factors, their effects don't simply add up they amplify each other. For example, if you have high total cholesterol and you smoke, you're at much greater risk than a nonsmoker with the same cholesterol level.

RISK FACTORS FOR CARDIOVASCULAR DISEASE TIED TO MENTAL DECLINE

Risk factors for cardiovascular disease may not only predict your chances of having a heart attack or stroke, but they may also anticipate how well you may think and remember as you age.

Scientists already knew that high blood pressure and diabetes could impair thinking abilities, but new research has identified two other cardiovascular risk factors that increased a person's chance of mental decline: obesity and smoking. Researchers from the University of Maine looked at data from the famed Framingham Heart Study, a well-know research project that has tracked the cardiovascular health of residents in a community near Boston for about fifty years.

A group of 1,799 participants between the age of fifty-five to eighty-five years took a series of eight neuropsychological tests designed to evaluate their thinking and memory abilities. Those who scored in the lowest 25 percent were labeled as "poor performers." After analyzing the total scores achieved on all eight tests, researchers discovered that those who had one of the four risk factors—obesity, smoking, hypertension, or diabetes—when they were tested had a 23 percent greater chance of being a "poor performers" when compared to those who had no risk factors. Each additional risk factor decreased mental function another 23 percent!

The researchers then narrowed their analysis to the scores on three tests that assessed learning and memory, excluding those that measured attention, concentration, or word fluency. As before, more risk factors translated into a higher chance of experiencing a mental decline. People with one risk factor averaged a 32 percent increased risk of mental decline over those with no risk factors, and again this chance increased by about 32 percent with each additional risk factor.

If you won't follow this plan for your heart, follow it for your mind. Lowering your risk for cardiovascular disease will not only help you live longer, but it will also increase your quality of life by preventing the mental decline that can accompany aging.

9

Fine-Tuning the Red Yeast Rice Diet

Cardiovascular disease can be complicated by a number of different conditions such as hypertension, syndrome X, homocysteinemia, and obesity. If you have any of these conditions, you need to do more than simply take red yeast rice. This chapter explains how to fine tune your diet and supplement regime if you have any of these complications.

HIGH BLOOD PRESSURE

High blood pressure, or hypertension, is a very difficult health disorder condition for a number of reasons.

- It is very common, affecting an estimated 24 percent of all American adults, about 43 million people. Among older adults the percentage is even higher.
- The affects of hypertension on tissues can be devastating. Not only does it accelerate atherosclerosis, but it

is a leading cause of strokes, kidney disease, and conges-
tive heart failure.

- Worst of all, hypertension does all this damage silently.
The victim feels no pain or discomfort. Typically, there
are no symptoms at all. When a victim does finally experience difficulties, the disease has already severely damaged tissues and vessels.

Hypertension is not a disease but a disorder. Once it is
established, it changes the structure of the arterioles—the small
muscular arteries. The smooth muscle cells in the arterial wall
multiply and enlarge so that the walls become thicker and the
opening becomes smaller. They also contract, further con-
stricting the opening. Think of your arteries as a garden hose.
When water comes out the end of the hose, it continues on for
an inch or two and then drops straight to the ground. You can't
water that bush at the other end of the garden with just a hose.
For that you need to attach a nozzle—a tube that is narrower
than the hose. When the water goes through the constricted
nozzle, it is under greater pressure. It shoots out the end, easily
reaching your bush ten feet away. And the narrower you make
your nozzle, the farther the water goes. Aim your nozzle at the
ground and it will move dirt and rocks with ease. It can also rip
away part of your lawn if you are not careful. When your
arteries constrict, your blood behaves like the water going
through the nozzle.

If the pressure in your arteries gets high enough, it too can
rip things. In this case, endothelial cells. High blood pressure
can peel the lining off artery walls and otherwise inflict
trauma on these delicate cells. There is no clear-cut threshold
of blood pressure above which damage occurs. The detrimental effects of hypertension increase continuously as pressure increases.

DIETARY RECOMMENDATIONS
FOR HYPERTENSION

It is very clear that diet affects blood pressure. Vegetarians, for example, tend to have lower blood pressures than nonvegetarians. When a group of people move from an area that has a low incidence of high blood pressure to one that has a high incidence of high blood pressure, they gradually assume the blood pressure incidence of the adopted area as they adopt the new diet.

Just how effective are diets in controlling blood pressure? The American Heart Association Nutrition Committee estimates that a reduction in diastolic blood pressure of just two millimeters of mercury (mm Hg) could lower a person's stroke risk by as much as 15 percent and lower heart disease risk by 6 percent.

HYPERTENSION AND SALT

A higher intake of salt is related to higher blood pressure, and there is good evidence that certain people with hypertension can lower their blood pressure by lowing their salt intake. If you suffer from high blood pressure, ask your physician if you are salt sensitive.

Americans eat much more salt than they need, and since I strongly believe that too much of anything is never a good idea, I recommend that everyone consume salt in moderation. A high intake of sodium is associated with more health problems than just hypertension. For the general population, the American Heart Association recommends that the average daily consumption of salt not exceed six grams daily. The DASH (Dietary Approaches to Stop Hypertension) diet below contains 7.5 grams in comparison to the standard American diet, which averages 10 mg. This is not difficult to achieve on a whole foods diet such as the Red Yeast Rice Diet since most salt is invisible—hidden inside of processed foods. When you avoid junk foods, you also avoid excess salt.

The sodium found in salt is not the only mineral implicated in hypertension. While Western diets contain too much sodium and chloride, they also contain too little of the other electrolyte minerals such as potassium, calcium, and magnesium. Several studies have shown that people who eat diets rich in potassium-containing foods tend to have lower blood pressure, while other studies have found this association in diets rich in calcium. Instead of blaming one mineral it might make more sense to consider hypertension a result of mineral imbalance.

THE DASH DIET

Rather than examine the effect of an individual nutrient or supplement, a group of researchers studied the impact of whole dietary patterns on blood pressure. The study group consisted of 459 adults with a starting blood pressure less than 160 mm Hg systolic and 80-95 mm Hg diastolic. Of those, 133 had high blood pressure and 326 had normal.

For the first three weeks volunteers ate the control diet, which was designed to imitate the average American diet. It was high in fat and low in fruits, vegetables, and dairy products. They were then randomly assigned to three groups. Each diet contained the same number of calories and amount of sodium.

- One group continued on the control diet.
- A second group ate a modified control diet that was similar to the control diet (high in fat) but provided nine to ten servings of fruits and vegetables and fewer sweets and snacks.

- A third group ate a combination diet—combination because it combined most of the characteristics that were thought to lower blood pressure. It contained less fat, saturated fat, and cholesterol, nine to ten servings of fruits and vegetables, and three servings of low-fat dairy foods.

After eight weeks blood pressures were again measured. When compared with the control diet, the combination diet significantly lowered both systolic and diastolic pressure while the fruit/vegetable diet lowered only systolic. The effect apparent within one week and was at its greatest and most stable at two weeks and after. Blood pressure reduction was greater in minority subjects when compared to nonminorities, but the difference was not statistically significant.

Subjects with high blood pressure showed a greater response than those with normal pressures. Among the 326 participants with normal blood pressure, the combination diet reduced systolic pressure by 3.5 mm Hg and diastolic blood pressure by an average of 2.1 mm Hg. But in the 133 participants with high blood pressure, the combination diet reduced systolic pressure 11.4 mm Hg and diastolic blood pressure 5.5 mm Hg. These results are similar to those seen with drug therapy, and the DASH research team has stated that their combination diet may be a good alternative to drug therapy for those subjects with Stage 1 hypertension.

If everyone adopted a DASH-type diet, it is estimated the incidence of coronary heart disease would fall by 15 percent and stroke by 27 percent! The Red Yeast Rice Diet is very similar to the combination diet. If you have hypertension and would like to duplicate the DASH diet, just add a few more servings of fruit and vegetables to the diet recommendation in Chapter 6. Make sure your mineral supplement contains potassium.

HYPERTENSION, STROKE, AND POTASSIUM

Diets rich in fruits, vegetables, and whole grain cereals may reduce a person's risk of stroke, especially in individuals with high blood pressure. Many researchers believe this is because the mineral content of the whole foods lowers blood pressure. A number of small studies suggested that a high intake of potassium in the diet could help reduce the risk of stroke. Researchers set out to determine whether these findings would still hold true in a larger study. They questioned 43,738 men who were part of the Health Professionals Follow-up Study, a dietary investigation of men who were free of heart disease and diabetes and who had not had a stroke. Of those, 8,520 had hypertension. During the eight-year study 328 individuals had strokes.

- Individuals in the top fifth of dietary potassium intake had a 38 percent lower risk of stroke than those in the bottom fifth. The major difference between the diets of the two groups was in their consumption of fruits and vegetables—about nine servings daily in the highest potassium group compared with four in the lowest.
- Individuals who had high blood pressure and who were also taking potassium supplements (about one gram per day) reduced their risk of stroke by 60 percent when compared to those with high blood pressure who weren't taking supplements.
- Men without high blood pressure whose diets were high in magnesium and cereal fiber also had a reduced risk of stroke when compared to men who ate lower levels of these nutrients.
- Those with high intakes of magnesium had a 30 percent decreased risk of stroke, and those with high intakes of

cereal fiber had a 40 percent decreased risk compared with those who ate low levels of these nutrients.

Other studies have shown that a high-potassium diet may reduce high blood pressure. In this case, however, the lower incidence of stroke did not seem to be caused by lower pressures. The differences in blood pressure were too small to cause such a dramatic decrease in stroke risk. Researchers concluded that there is strong support for a stroke-preventive effect from diets rich in potassium, magnesium, and cereal fiber. This was found to be particularly true in individuals with high blood pressure, further suggesting that high-potassium diets might be beneficial in this segment of the population.

Diet Tips for Hypertension

- Choose fruits and vegetables that are rich in potassium, magnesium, and calcium. Food sources of these minerals can be found in Chapter 7.
- Reduce the amount of caffeine and sugar in your diet. Both can increase the amount of potassium that is excreted by the kidney.
- Supplement your diet with a comprehensive mineral supplement that contains calcium, magnesium, and potassium.
- Take an arginine supplement, one to two grams in divided doses on an empty stomach.
- Eat fatty fish at least twice a week and take a fish oil supplement with it.

LESS SALT, FEWER STROKES

Research has shown that the risk of having a stroke increases as blood pressure increases. Research has also shown that drug treatment can decrease the incidence of stroke. Recently a study done by St. George's Hospital Medical School found that a modest reduction in salt intake was just as effective in lowering blood pressure than treatment with diuretics such as thiazides.

This English study looked at forty-seven volunteers aged sixty to seventy-eight years with a blood pressure range of 123-205 mm Hg systolic and 64-112 mm Hg diastolic. A diet low in salt—five grams a day—was compared to a diet high in salt—ten grams a day. Participants with both high blood pressure and normal pressure experienced a decrease in blood pressure. The average reduction was 7.2 mm Hg systolic and 3.2 mm Hg diastolic. This was estimated to correspond to a 36 percent reduction in stroke risk over a five-year period!

The researchers concluded that the decrease in blood pressure achievable through a low-salt diet could result in a major reduction in the incidence of strokes. What is important is that the reduction in salt intake was accomplished simply by not cooking with salt, adding salt at the table, and avoiding salted junk foods.

How to Reduce Salt Intake

To achieve no more than 2,400 mg/day of sodium, choose foods that are naturally low in salt, like fresh fruits and vegetables. Limit excessively salty foods: smoked, cured, or processed meat; some convenience foods like frozen meals and regular canned soups; certain spices like regular soy sauce, garlic salt, and other salted condiments; highly salted snacks like salted crackers, chips, pretzels, popcorn, and nuts; and many sauces, mixes and "instant" products. Break the habit of adding salt to food or water during cooking or at the table. Use herbs, spices, and fruit juices in place of salt to season food, and rinse canned vegetables to remove excess salt. Read the nutrition label on food packages to select foods lower in sodium.

AFRICAN AMERICANS AND HYPERTENSION

In the United States, rates of heart disease, hypertension, diabetes, and obesity are higher among African Americans, particularly African American women. High blood pressure develops earlier in African Americans when compared to Caucasian

Americans. Average blood pressures are much higher too. According to a report issued by the National Heart, Lung and Blood Institute (part of the National Institutes of Health), this translates into an 80 percent higher rate of death from stroke, a 50 percent higher rate of death from heart disease, and a 320 percent greater rate of hypertension-related end-stage renal disease than those in the general population.

Researchers from Meharry Medical College and Vanderbilt University wanted to know if these differences were due to genetics or lifestyle. To answer this question, they studied the nutrition and exercise habits of 223 members of the African Hebrew Israelite community, a group of African Americans who had emigrated in the early 1970s from the United States to Israel. This group was of interest because they are the first group of African Americans that has actually emigrated from America in large numbers and changed their entire lifestyle.

The group had virtually no health problems despite the fact that 43 percent reported a family history of hypertension and/or coronary artery disease. Questionnaires showed that they had a vegan diet (eat no meat or animal products), and more than 80 percent reported at least one session of exercise per week with 53 percent reporting three or more exercise sessions per week. Participants also did not use tobacco and reported no alcohol or drug abuse.

The research team concluded that African Americans are not necessarily genetically predisposed to hypertension and that hypertension, obesity, and high cholesterol can be prevented with a drastic change in lifestyle.

ARGININE AND HYPERTENSION

Constricted arteries are dilated by nitric oxide, also called endothelial-derived relaxing factor. You cannot supplement nitric oxide, but you can take arginine, an amino acid that is a precursor to the enzyme that produces it. By increasing arginine you produce more enzyme and therefore more nitric oxide. Arginine supplementation has been shown to reduce blood pressure. Since lysine, another amino acid, competes for absorption with arginine, do not take the two together. Supplementing lysine can also cause a decrease in arginine for the same reason.

In Chapter 8 we talked about how to measure your blood pressure. If your pressures are elevated, see your physician for guidance and make sure that your have your blood pressure monitored on a regular basis. Hypertension can occur alone or in conjunction with insulin resistance syndrome, a condition the often precedes diabetes.

DIABETES

Approximately 16 million Americans have diabetes, and type 2 diabetes accounts for nearly 95 percent of all diagnosed cases. It costs the United States $98 billion each year, more than AIDS and breast cancer combined. More than 15 million Americans are thought to suffer from adult-onset diabetes, which typically develops after age forty. It is estimated that half of those afflicted do not even know they have the disease.

People with diabetes often develop cardiovascular complications. Recent research indicates that poor control of blood sugar levels correlates with the incidence of coronary heart disease, peripheral arterial disease (claudication), and amputations of the lower extremities. Hyperglycemia has been linked to hypertension in several studies. Researchers now believe that all diabetes complications are caused by elevated blood sugar levels, which may be prevented or reduced by improved control of blood sugar.

Insulin is a hormone secreted by the pancreas in response to a meal that contains carbohydrates. It regulates energy production by helping the glucose molecules to enter hungry cells. After you eat, the glucose from your meal enters your bloodstream and glucose levels rise. This stimulates the release of insulin from the pancreas, and insulin levels rise in proportion to the glucose levels. Insulin must then attach itself to an insulin receptor in order for the glucose to be carried into the cell. In this way insulin is like a key that must fit into a keyhole or receptor for the glucose "door" to open.

People with type 1 diabetes have had their insulin producing cells in the pancreas destroyed so they make no insulin. When there is a lack of insulin, it is like having no keys and cells die of starvation while surrounded by food. Glucose levels in the blood rise (a condition called high blood sugar or hyperglycemia), and the person develops type 1 diabetes.

Sometimes insulin is plentiful, but the glucose still cannot enter the cells because of defective insulin receptors on the cells. This is like having keys but no keyholes or keyholes of the wrong shape. This can happen in people who have type 2 diabetes (adult-onset). The cells are said to be insulin resistant since they resist the action of insulin. The insulin cannot enter the cells, and it builds up in the blood causing a condition called hyperinsulinemia (high blood insulin levels). Glucose levels also rise causing hyperglycemia (high blood sugar levels). Constant exposure of the arterial walls to insulin can damage the endothelial cells, initiating atherosclerosis. In the subendothelial space, insulin can stimulate smooth muscle cells to grow and promote the development of plaque. This is why 50 to 60 percent of all deaths in diabetics are from cardiovascular diseases with coronary heart disease the cause of 40 to 50 percent of those deaths.

Supplements for Diabetics

- Arginine: one to two grams a day, taken in divided doses on an empty stomach
- Fish oil: 1,800 mg of EPA and 1,200 mg of DHA as fish oil.
- Chromium: This should be included in your mineral supplement. Check the label to make sure you are getting 100 percent of the RDA.
- Magnesium: Part of your intake should come from your mineral supplement. Avoid supplements that contain the entire RDA in one pill; your body cannot absorb all that magnesium at once. Ideally you should take a calcium and magnesium citrate and/or malate twice a day in addition to the amount you are getting in your mineral supplement. Make sure that you are getting at least 1,200 mg of calcium a day and 300 mg of magnesium.

FISH OILS AND FIBER BENEFIT DIABETICS

Numerous studies have shown that fish oil supplementation lowers the levels of VLDL and triglycerides but has little effect on LDL levels and total cholesterol. There were also some reports that supplementation with fish oil may worsen blood sugar control. This led researchers at Case Western Reserve University to test a regime of soluble fiber and fish oil. Their experiment involved fifteen nonobese type 2 diabetic patients aged thirty-two to seventy-four years. The patients continued their usual diabetic diet and medication during the entire study period. For the first four weeks the patients were fed 20 grams of fish oil each day. During the next four weeks all patients received the fish oil plus 15 grams/day of soluble apple pectin.

- Fish oil supplementation alone lowered the levels of tri-acylglycerol by 41 percent and VLDL cholesterol by 36 percent.

- When apple pectin was added, triglyceride and VLDL cholesterol levels were both lowered by 38 percent. Total cholesterol levels also decreased by 13 percent and LDL cholesterol by 7 percent. There was no significant change in HDL cholesterol level.

The researchers concluded that a combination of fish oil supplementation and increased fiber intake (up to 40 grams/day total) may be a beneficial addition to the conventional treatment of high cholesterol levels in type 2 diabetics.

CHROMIUM

Chromium is a trace mineral involved in glucose metabolism as part of the glucose tolerance factor (GTF). It helps with the absorption of insulin and to keep glucose levels even. Chromium levels are low in the average American, not a surprise since the best sources of chromium are whole grains. Low chromium levels are also more common in patients who have heart disease. Vanadium and manganese are two other trace minerals that are involved in glucose metabolism. Check your mineral supplement to make sure that all three are included.

Sources of Chromium:

- Acidic foods cooked in stainless steel pots
- Black pepper
- Broccoli
- Hard water
- High chromium brewer's yeast
- Molasses
- Potato skins
- Poultry
- Thyme
- Wheat germ
- Whole grains

MAGNESIUM AND DIABETES

Low levels of magnesium in your blood may mean you are at risk to develop type 2 diabetes—if you are white. Several short-term studies had looked at high doses of magnesium as treatment for diabetes. The magnesium was able to improve the body's ability to handle glucose.

Investigators at the Johns Hopkins University School of Medicine measured magnesium levels in 12,398 nondiabetic, middle-aged African American and white subjects and followed them for six years. By the end of the study, there were 807 new cases of type 2 diabetes, and whites, those with the lowest level of magnesium at the beginning of the study, were at the greatest risk (94 percent) for developing type 2 diabetes during the study. No association was found between magnesium levels and the development of diabetes in African Americans.

No one knows how this magnesium deficiency causes diabetes. The authors of this study hypothesized that because magnesium is involved in carbohydrate and insulin metabolism, low magnesium levels may impair these processes, which could eventually lead to diabetes development. You can increase your magnesium levels by eating more of the magnesium-rich foods found in Chapter 7. Your mineral supplement should also contain magnesium.

ARGININE MAY PROTECT AGAINST HYPERGLYCEMIA

In an Italian study, researchers at the University of Naples linked hyperglycemia to several other important risk factors for heart disease. The participants were twenty healthy, nonobese twenty-eight-year-olds. They were given an injection of glucose followed by a 30 percent glucose infusion to keep blood sugar levels elevated for ninety minutes. Researchers found that the glucose increased blood pressure and heart rate and significantly decreased blood flow to the legs. Platelet aggregation, blood thickness, and the level of plasma catecholamines—epinephrine and norepinephrine—also increased significantly.

In a separate experiment, the researchers infused L-arginine, an amino acid, into the bloodstream during the last thirty minutes of the glucose infusion. This resulted in a rapid fall in blood pressure levels, a restoration of blood flow to the legs, and a significant decrease in platelet aggregation and blood viscosity. Heart rate and plasma catecholamine levels were not modified by the L-arginine infusion.

The researchers concluded that hyperglycemia may independently contribute to the development of cardiovascular complications in diabetes patients and that L-arginine can reverse them. You can buy arginine supplements in your health food store.

We do not have room here to list all of the dietary treatments for diabetes. However, the goal of your diet should be to keep your blood sugar levels even and under control. This will reduce your risk of cardiovascular disease and other complications. Invest in a few sessions with a dietician or licensed nutritionist for guidance in planning your meals. You may have to take a medicine if diet alone does not work.

INSULIN RESISTANCE SYNDROME

You don't have to have diabetes for your cells to be insulin resistant. You could have a condition called the insulin resistance syndrome, or syndrome X. High insulin levels is just one of a group of symptoms that seem to occur together in this syndrome. If the symptoms in Table 9-1 are familiar, you might have a faulty glucose metabolism.

Table 9-1: Syndrome X

Some risk factors for heart disease seem to cluster together. These risk factors include:

- High blood pressure
- A combination of high triglycerides, low HDL cholesterol, and the presence of small LDL particles
- Central fat distribution. Excess fat is more often deposited centrally around the trunk and less often on hips, arms, and legs. This is sometimes referred to as the "apple shape." You do not have to be overweight to have this shape. It's the pattern of fat storage rather than the obesity that is linked to the syndrome.
- Impaired glucose tolerance. Glucose intolerance refers to a condition in which blood sugar levels are higher than normal but not high enough to be classified as diabetes (between 140 to 199 mg/dl in a two-hour oral glucose tolerance test). About 11 percent of adults are glucose intolerant and 40 to 45 percent of persons over the age of sixty-five are either glucose intolerant or have noninsulin dependent diabetes mellitus (NIDDM).
- Insulin resistance. Insulin resistance describes a condition in which insulin is unable to enter the tissues. The tissues are "resistant to insulin." This results in high levels of circulating insulin. Insulin can damage the vessel wall.

In order to understand the role of hyperinsulinemia as a risk factor for cardiovascular disease, Finnish researchers studied a group of 970 healthy men (who did not have cardiovascular disease or diabetes) for a twenty-two-year period. During that time 164 of them had a heart attack.

At the first five-year follow-up, the scientists discovered that participants with the highest levels of insulin were more than three times as likely to have a heart attack as those with the lowest levels of insulin. At the ten-year follow-up, those with the highest insulin levels were at 2.7 times greater risk than those at the lowest levels. Researchers concluded that hyperinsulinemia was just as good as cholesterol levels when predicting who would develop cardiovascular disease. In fact, when compared to other risk factors, insulin levels were the most statistically significant predictor of heart attack risk found during the study. Other factors that predicted cardiovascular disease include high blood pressure, as the participants in the study grew older, and smoking.

DIETARY MODIFICATIONS
FOR SYNDROME X

If this profile fits you, what can you do? The most effective treatment for syndrome X is dietary. By following the Red Yeast Rice Diet you have already greatly decreased the amount of refined foods that you eat. These refined foods can elevate glucose and insulin levels. You have already increased your vitamin C content, which will help to keep glucose production by the liver at normal levels. Dutch researchers at the National Institute of Public Health found that one ounce of fish (lean, fatty, or canned) protected against the development of glucose tolerance.

You can help keep your blood sugar and insulin levels even by increasing the time food spends in your stomach and by decreasing the rate at which carbohydrate foods are digested. For example, both fat and fiber will slow gastric emptying. This allows only small amounts of sugar to enter your bloodstream at a time, reducing hyperglycemia. It also reduces the magnitude of the insulin response, reducing hyperinsulinemia. If you shown signs of insulin resistance, try these tips.

- Eat only brown rice, brown bread, and whole grains. Not only are these sources of chromium, they contain fiber that will increase the time food spends in your stomach.
- Choose whole fruits and vegetables over fruit and sweet vegetable juices. An apple will only slightly increase insulin levels when compared to the rise induced by a glass of apple juice.
- Don't eat sweet foods on an empty stomach. The stomach quickly empties and the sugar is immediately absorbed. Drink sweet juices and eat fruits on a full stomach that contains some fat.
- Don't overcook your pasta dishes or the starches will enter your blood too fast. Cook pasta only until it is al dente.
- Use generous amounts of apple pie spices: cinnamon, cloves, bay, and turmeric. These spices and tuna fish and peanut butter were shown to contain an unidentified insulin potentiating factor that improves glucose tolerance.
- Consume foods rich in chromium.
- Exercise. Moderate aerobic exercise has been shown repeatedly to improve insulin resistance, reduce hypertension, and improve HDL/LDL ratios.

HOMOCYSTEINEMIA

Is it possible that a vitamin B deficiency could cause heart disease? According to Cleveland researchers, as much as one-fifth of the U.S. population may be at increased risk of heart attacks and strokes because they do not get enough vitamin B6 (pyridoxine) and folic acid. The Cleveland study, part of the

European Concerted Action Project, examined 750 people with atherosclerosis or blockages in the blood vessels of the heart, brain, and leg. A control group of 800 healthy individuals of similar age and sex was also included. They found that those with a pyridoxine deficiency were almost twice as likely to have heart disease and stroke than those without such a deficiency. The association of a pyridoxine and folic acid deficiency with heart disease and stroke may be connected to their role in homocysteine metabolism.

Homocysteine is an amino acid that is part of the methionine metabolism. Methionine is converted to homocysteine which is then immediately changed into cysteine by an enzyme that requires pyridoxine. The reaction also goes backwards; homocysteine can also be recycled back into methionine with the help of folic acid. Normally homocysteine exists only for a brief time. However, if not enough pyridoxine or folate is present, or if the enzymes do not work as they should, the reaction is not always completed and some homocysteine remains and accumulates.

This accumulated homocysteine has been shown to be toxic, oxidizing both the endothelial membranes and LDL particles. High levels of blood homocysteine are present in an estimated 20 million Americans or more than one of every three people with cardiovascular disease.

One of the surprises of this study was that vitamin B6 deficiency was still linked to heart disease and stroke in study participants who had normal levels of homocysteine. Pyridoxine may make the blood more prone to the formation of thrombi (blood clots) that can obstruct blood vessels or alter levels of cholesterol.

Folic acid is also necessary in early pregnancy to prevent birth defects in the embryo's neural tube, which develops into the brain and spinal cord. Neural tube defects can result in debilitating conditions that last a lifetime, such as spina bifida. Because of the importance of folic acid in the diet, the FDA recently increased its folic acid recommendation from 180 micrograms to 400 micrograms for adults and from 400 micrograms to 800 micrograms for pregnant women. It has also mandated that folic acid be added to foods such as flour beginning in 1998.

DIETARY RECOMMENDATIONS FOR HOMOCYSTEINEMIA

When the American Heart Association Nutrition Committee met in November 1998, they announced that homocysteine is "worthy of consideration by the press, the American public, and the world." They added that homocysteine is a potential non-traditional risk factor and that "diet is a major controlling factor for blood levels of homocysteine." Take extra care to assure that your diet contains enough of the B vitamins. This condition is a sign that your present diet is inadequate. Folic acid is water soluble so it will leach out of foods into the cooking water. Prolonged heating or boiling also reduces the folic acid content of foods. To protect the folic acid content of your food, steam your vegetables lightly.

Brewer's yeast, fortified cereals, nuts, and legumes are good sources of both nutrients, and more sources for folic acid and pyridoxine can be found in Chapter 7. Make sure that your vitamin regime contains at least 400 mcg of folic acid, 10 mg of pyridoxine, and 400 mcg of vitamin B12. Although B12 is also involved in methionine metabolism, it is often recommended because some experts are afraid folate supplementation may mask a B12 deficiency. The newest nutrient to achieve vitamin status is choline. Like folic acid, choline is involved in metabolizing homocysteine and has been shown to be partially effective in lowering homocysteine levels in humans. Lecithin, or phosphatidylcholine, is a good source of choline. It is the natural emulsifier found in egg yolks. Other research suggests lecithin protects the heart by affecting the way the body handles cholesterol.

Can fortified cereal products have an effect on homocysteine levels? To answer this question researchers conducted a fifteen-week randomized double-blind, placebo-controlled clinical trial in which participants were given 3/4 cup of Total cereal each day. Total breakfast cereal is fortified with 100 percent of the Daily Value of folic acid. The treatment group lowered their blood levels of homocysteine by an average of 11 percent. The study was published in the *New England Journal of Medicine*.

OBESITY

When an individual takes in more energy than he or she uses, he or she is said to be in positive energy balance. This is fine if the person in question is still growing, pregnant, or recovering from an illness, but if you are a healthy nonpregnant adult, a constant energy surplus results in a slow weight gain. This can be avoided by either eating fewer calories or by burning more calories. I recommend you do a little of both. A sedentary lifestyle is another risk factor for cardiovascular disease.

The National Health and Nutrition Examination Survey III, taken between 1988 and 1994, indicated that 22.5 percent of men and women between the ages twenty and seventy-four were obese. If our definition of obesity is broadened to include people who are overweight, over 50 percent of American adults are overweight today. Obesity contributes to more than 300,000 deaths each year with health care costs amounting to nearly $70 billion per year. You can determine if you are overweight by following the instructions in Chapter 8 for weight evaluation. There you will find formulas for calculating your IBW (ideal body weight), BMI (body mass index), and waist-to-hip ratio.

If you fit the definition of obese, do your best to lose at least 10 to 20 percent of your weight. This is especially important if you have an "apple" shape—and store your fat in your abdomen. Forget about dieting all the way down to your ideal body weight. In most cases it is not necessary.

Why worry if you are obese?

- Obesity is associated with type 2 diabetes. Eighty percent of diabetics are more than 20 percent overweight. Weight loss improves glucose tolerance, and in some cases the diabetes resolves.
- Obesity is associated with hypertension. When overweight hypertensives reduce their weight, they also reduce their blood pressure.
- Obesity is associated with high LDL levels. Even a small weight loss enhances the LDL-cholesterol reduction achieved by reducing intakes of saturated fat and cholesterol. For example, five to ten pounds of weight loss can double the LDL-cholesterol reduction achieved by reducing saturated fat and cholesterol.

The Red Yeast Rice Diet was not designed to be a weight loss diet. However, if you are now eating a lot of processed foods, animal products, and sweets, this diet will result in a modest weight loss. It may be all the diet you need.

WEIGHT REDUCTION AND EXERCISE

Regular exercise is one of the most important actions you can take to prevent heart disease, stroke, hypertension, obesity, and diabetes. It goes hand and hand with diet; your body needs both to keep healthy. There is no substitute for vigorous exercise just as there is no substitute for good food. The more active you are, the more weight you will lose. The more weight you lose, the greater your LDL reduction and HDL increase. Weight-bearing exercise is important for building and keeping bone density, thereby preventing osteoporosis. Exercise can even help to reduce insulin resistance and prevent diabetes. It will also do wonders for your mental health. There is no better stress reliever than exercise.

- A British study found that in middle-aged men, the risk of heart attack and stroke can be decreased by over 50 percent simply by walking regularly and participating once a week in a recreational activity or sport.
- If postmenopausal women take a thirty to forty-five minute walk three times a week, they will cut their risk of a heart attack in half.
- Men and women who exercise at least once a week lower their risk of developing diabetes by 30 percent.
- Find an aerobic exercise you enjoy. This includes running, jogging, biking, cross country skiing, and even vigorous walking. If you don't like your exercise program, you are not going to keep with it, so put some thought into choosing activities.
- Start slowly and build. Gradually increase how long you spend exercising until you reach thirty to forty-five minutes at least three times a week. The higher your level of exercise the greater your weight loss and health benefits. If you are obese or have been inactive for many years, it may take months before you can exercise this much. That's OK. Just take it slow and don't quit.
- Be persistent and don't get discouraged. Find a friend, or join an exercise group, to keep you motivated and committed to exercise. I like to walk, but rainy Washington State prevents me from going outdoors during the winter months. I solved this by buying a treadmill. It sits right in front of a TV so I can walk and watch at the same time.

How to Order
Red Yeast Rice

If you cannot find red yeast rice at a health food store close to you, it is available through mail order, direct sales, and the Internet. The premier brand of red yeast rice is Cholestin, manufactured by Pharmanex. This is the brand used in almost all of the research studies. The other companies here also sell standardized red yeast rice. If you buy a cheap brand of red yeast rice that does not lower your cholesterol, it may be that particular product that does not work rather than red yeast rice itself. Try one of the following brands. If you find an effective brand of red yeast rice that is not listed here, please contact me so I can include it in later editions.

PHARMANEX INC.
Most of the research on red yeast rice was done using Cholestin, a high-quality red yeast rice product made by Pharmanex, a Simi, California, company. Pharmanex makes a variety of botanical products in addition to Cholestin. Pharmanex is owned by NuSkin, which also markets IDN products—Interior Design Nutritionals. Cholestin is available through all IDN representatives.

To learn more about the Pharmanex line of natural health care products or to order, call Pharmanex customer service at:

Phone: (800) 800-0260
Fax: (800) 800-0259
Internet orders: www.pharmanex.com

Or write:
Pharmanex
73 West Center
Provo, Utah 84601

PHARM N SEAS

This California company makes three products that contain red yeast rice extract. All contain 9.6 mg of HMG-CoA reductase inhibitors. According to a Pharm N Seas representative, its products are analyzed to make sure they contain the advertised levels of active ingredients.

- Heartrol (a single capsule a day of red yeast rice formula)
- C-HC (a single capsule formula for elevated cholesterol *and* homocysteine)
- Advanced Heart (red yeast rice extract, CoQ10, and beta sitosterol)

You can order all Pharm N Seas products through a variety of sources including selected health food stores, or you can contact them directly at:

Phone orders: (888) 545-7327
Fax: (949) 461-3953

Or write:
Pharm N Seas
24831 Alicia Parkway, Suite C-166
Laguna Hills, CA 92653

SEACOAST NATURAL FOODS
Seacoast Natural Foods sell Pharm N Seas products, including red yeast rice. To order Seacoast products:

Phone: (877) 229-1779
Fax: (619) 429-1770
E-mail: seacoop@seacoastvitamins.com
Internet orders: www.seacoast.com

Or write:
Seacoast Natural Foods
600 Palm Avenue #106
Imperial Beach, CA 91932

Questions and information: (800) 555-6792
Business Hours (Pacific time):
Monday–Friday: 9:00 A.M. to 9:00 P.M.
Saturday–Sunday: 9:00 A.M. to 8:00 P.M.

RICH NATURE LABS
Rich Nature Labs is a Washington State company. It sells and makes CholesCare—made from a proprietary strain of standard-ized *Monascus purpureus* Went yeast. Rich Nature's CholesCare contains a higher percentage of HMG-CoA reductase inhibitors (0.5% per capsule) than other brands (0.4% per capsule).

If you order more than $20.00 per order, shipping is free.

To order CholesCare:
Phone: (206) 547-4248
Fax: (206) 547-7935
Email: info@richnature.com
Internet orders: www.richnature.com

Or write:
Rich Nature Labs, Inc.
4000 Aurora North, Suite 100
Seattle, WA 98103

TO ORDER THE FIBER SUPPLEMENTS MENTIONED IN CHAPTER 7

Fiber Plan is available from the Shaklee Corp. It is available as a flavored and unflavored drink mix, tablets, and crunch topping. Shaklee manufactures a wide variety of vitamins and minerals, herbal medicines, sport and fitness products, weight management aids, and natural skin care items.

To find a distributor near you:

- Call 1 (800) 848-2532 or 1 (800) VITA LEA
- Internet: http://www.shaklee.com/
- look in yellow or white pages under Shaklee Distributors

VITAMIN RESEARCH COMPANY

Although this company does not presently sell red yeast rice products, it does offer other quality products, and as the market expands it may offer red yeast rice formulas. Call for a catalogue and free four-month subscription to its monthly newsletter.

Phone: (800) 877-2447
Fax: (800) 877-3292
Internet orders: www.vrp.com

Or write:
Vitamin Research Products Inc
3579 Hwy 50 East
Carson City, NV 89701

LIFE EXTENSION FOUNDATION (ALSO SELLS SUPPLEMENTS)
Call for a free directory of nutrients or to order:

Phone: (800) 841-5433
Internet orders: www.lef.org

Or write:
Life Extension Foundation
PO Box 229120
Hollywood, FL 33022-9120

CFIDS AND FIBROMYAGIA HEALTH RESOURCE
The CFIDS and Fibromyagia Health Resource sells its own brand of vitamins and minerals at very reasonable prices. Free shipping on orders over $50 or frequent sales. Sends a free catalog on request.

Phone: (800) 366-6056
Internet orders: www.immunesupport.com

Or write:
1187 Coast Village Road, #1-280
Santa Barbara, CA 93108-2794

References

CHAPTER 1

Dai Y, Luo X. 1996. "Functional food in China." *Nutrition Reviews* 54: S21–S23.

Endo A. 1979. "Monacolin K, a new hypercholesterolemic agent produced by a *Monascus* species." *Journal of Antibiotics* (Tokyo) 32: 852–4.

Endo A., M. Kuroda, and Y. Tsujita. 1976. "ML-236A, ML-236B, and ML-236C, new inhibitors of cholesterolgenesis produced by Penicillium citrinum." *Journal of Antibiotics* (Tokyo) 29: 1346–8.

Kennedy, A., and K. Auclair, et. al. 1999. "Modulation of polyketide synthase activity by accessory proteins during lovastatin biosynthesis." *Science* 284: 1368–1372.

Mei, F. 1990. Red yeast flavored duck. From Fang Mei, *Illustrated Cookbook of Regional Chinese Cuisine*. Guangxi, China: Guangxi National Press. 177-88.

Weng, Weijian, M.D., and Junshi Chen, M.D. 1996. "The Eastern perspective on functional foods based on traditional Chinese medicine." *Nutrition Reviews* 54: S11–S16.

CHAPTER 3

Buring, J. E., and C. H. Hennekens. 1997. "Antioxidant vitamins and cardiovascular disease." *Nutrition Reviews* 55: S53–60.

Chan, A. C. 1998. "Vitamin E and atherosclerosis." *Journal of Nutrition* 128: 1593–96.

Dietschy, J. M. 1997. "Theoretical considerations of what regulates low-density-lipoprotein and high-density-lipoprotein cholesterol." *American Journal of Clinical Nutrition* 65: 1581S–9S.

Hornstra, G., C.A. Barth, R. P. Mesink, M. Mutanin, et. al. 1998. "Functional food science and the cardiovascular system." *British Food Science* 80: S113–46.

Luc, G., and J. C. Fruchart. 1991. "Oxidation of lipoproteins and atherosclerosis." *American Journal of Clinical Nutrition* 53: 206S–9S.

Staprans, I., J. H. Rapp, Pan Xian-Mang, D. A. Hardman, and K. R. Feingold. 1996. "Oxidized lipids in the diet accelerate lipid deposition in the arteries of cholesterol-fed rabbits." *Arterioscleo Thromb Vasc Biology* 16: 533–38.

Staprans, I., P. Xian-Mang, J. H. Rapp, and K. R. Feingold. "Oxidized cholesterol in the diet accelerates the development of aortic atherosclerosis in cholesterol-fed rabbits." *Arterioscleo Thromb Vasc Biology* 1998 18: 977–83.

CHAPTER 4

Anderson, J. W., D. A. Deakins, T. L. Floore, F. M. Smith, and S. E. Whitis. "Dietary fiber and coronary heart disease." *Critical Reviews in Food Science and Nutrition* 29: 95–135.

Adler, Adam J., and Bruce J. Holub. 1997. "Effect of garlic and fish-oil supplementation on serum lipid and lipoprotein concentrations in hypercholesterolemic men." *American Journal of Clinical Nutrition* 65: 445–50.

Harris, W. S. 1997. "n-3 Fatty acids and serum lipoproteins: human studies." *America Journal of Clinical Nutrition* 65 (supplement): 1645–54.

Raper, N. R., F. J. Cronin, and J. Exler. 1992. "Omega three fatty acid content of the US food supply." *Journal of the American College of Nutrition* 11: 304–308.

Steiner, Manfred, et al. 1996. "A double-blind crossover study in moderately hypercholesterolemic men that compared the effect of aged garlic extract and placebo administration on blood lipids." *American Journal of Clinical Nutrition* 64: 866-70.–

Chapter 5

Beijing Institute of Clinical Pharmacology. Acute toxicity experiment of XueZhiKang in mice. Unpublished.

Beijing Institute of Clinical Pharmacology. Long-term toxicity studies in animals. Red Yeast Experimental Report. Unpublished by Lee Changling.

Byington, R. P., J. W. Jukema, J. T. Salonen, B. Pitt, A. V. Bruschke, H. Hoen, et. al. 1995. "Reduction in cardiovascular events during pravastatin therapy. Pooled analysis of clinical events of the Pravastatin. Atherosclerosis Intervention Program." *Circulation* 92: 2419–25.

Changling, Li. Acute toxicity studies in animals. Red Yeast Experimental Report. Dept. of Pharmacology, Beijing Medical University.

Changling, Li. XueZhiKang capsule long-term toxicity experiment. Dept of Pharmacology, Beijing Medical University.

Downs, J. R., M. Clearfield, S. Weis, et. al. 1998. "Primary prevention of acute coronary events with Lovastatin in men and women with average cholesterol levels." *Journal of the American Medical Association* 279: 1615–22.

Drug Topics Natural Products Update. June 1997.

Frick, M. H., O. Elo, K. Haapa, O. P. Heinonen, P. Heinsalmi, P. Helo, et al. 1987. "Helsinki Heart Study: primary-prevention trial with Gemfibrozil in middle-aged men with dyslipidemia. Safety of treatment, changes in risk factors, and incidence of coronary heart disease." *New England Journal of Medicine* 317: 1237–45.

Havel, R. 1999. "Dietary supplement or drug? The case of Cholestin." *American Journal of Clinical Nutrition* vol 69: 175–6.

Heber, D., I. Yip, J. M. Ashley, D. A. Elashoff, V. L.W. Go. 1999. "Cholesterol-lowering effects of a proprietary Chinese red yeast rice dietary supplement." *American Journal of Clinical Nutrition* 69: 231–6.

Li, C., Y. Zhu, Y. Wang, J. Zhu, J. Chang, and D. Kritchevsky. 1998. "*Monascus Purpureus*-fermented rice (red yeast rice): a natural food product that lowers blood cholesterol in animal models of hypercholesterolemia." *Nutrition Research* 18: 71–81.

Liu, A., L. Zhao, Y. Ahang, et. al. 1996. "Clinical observation of treatment of hyperlipidemia with Xuezhikang." *Chinese Medical News* 11: 12–13.

Perreault, S., V. H. Hamilton, F. Lavoie, S. Grover. 1998. "Treating hyperlipidemia for the primary prevention of coronary disease: are higher does of lovastatin cost-effective?" *Archives of Internal Medicine* 159: 375–81.

Scandinavian Simvastatin Survival Study Group (4S). 1994. *Lancet* 344: 1383–1389.

Scandinavian Simvastatin Survival Study Group. 1994. "Randomized trial of cholesterol lowering in 4,444 patients with coronary heart disease: the Scandinavian Simvastatin Survival Study (4S)." *Lancet* 344: 1383–9.

Shen, Z., P. Yu, M. Sun, et. al. 1996. "A prospective study on Zhitai capsule in the treatment of primary hyperlipidemia." *National Medical Journal of China* 76: 156–7.

Su, M., X. Wang, Y. Li, and Z. Gao. 1995. "A clinical trial of Xuezhikang capsule in the treatment of hyperlipidemia." *New Chinese Herbal Medicine Clinical Pharmacology* 6: 13–16.

Wang, J., L. Zongliang, C. Jiamin, W. Want, W. Meizhe Kou, et. al. 1997. "Multicenter clinical trial of the serum lipid-lowering effects of a *Monascus purpureus* (red yeast) rice preparation from traditional Chinese medicine." *Current Therapeutic Research* 58

Wang, J., M. Su, Z. Lu, et. al. 1995. "Clinical trial of extract of *Monascus purpureus* (red yeast) in the treatment of hyper-lipidemia." *Chin Journal Exp Ther Prep Chin Med* 12: 1–5.

Xie, S, and Z. Duan. 1996. "Xuezhikang capsule regulates blood lipids with high efficacy: an overview of its prepara-tion, pharmacology, toxicology, and results of clinical trials." *Chinese Medical News* 11: 13–14.

CHAPTER 6

Archer, S. L., D. Green, M. Chamberlain, A. R. Dyer, and K. Liu. 1994. "Association of dietary fish and n-3 fatty acid intake with hemostatic factor in the coronary artery risk development in young adults." (CARDIA) Study.

Dreher, M. L., and C. V. Maher. 1996. "The traditional and emerging role of nuts in healthful diets." *Nutrition Reveiws* 54:241–45.

Schaefer, E. J. 1993. "New recommendations for the diagnosis and treatment of plasma lipid abnormalities." *Nutrition Reviews* 51: 246–52.

CHAPTER 7

Kantola, Teemu, M.D., Kari T. Kivisto, M.D., and Pertti J. Neuvonen, M.D. 1998. "Grapefruit juice greatly increases serum concentrations of lovastatin and lovastatin acid." *Clin Pharmacol Ther* (Helsinki) 63: 397–402.

Urgert, R., and M. B. Katan. 1997. "The cholesterol-raising factor from coffee beans." *Annual Review of Nutrition* 17: 305–24.

CHAPTER 9

Khan, A., N. A. Bryden, M. M. Polansky, and R. A. Anderson. 1990. "Insulin potentiating factor and chromium content in selected foods and spices." *Biological Trace Element Research* 24: 183–88.

Index